Clinics in Developmental Medicine No. 29

The Infant Cry

A Spectrographic and Auditory Analysis

O. Wasz-Höckert, J. Lind, V. Vuorenkoski, T. Partanen and E. Valanne

Department of Pediatrics, University of Oulu, Oulu, Finland; Wenner-Gren Cardiovascula Research Laboratory, Nortull's Hospital, Stockholm, Sweden; Karolinska Institute, Stockholm Sweden.

Preface

Ronald Illingworth

35s. or $4.50

1968

Spastics International Medical Publications in Association with William Heinemann Medical Books Ltd.

SBN 433-34880-1

Printed in England at THE LAVENHAM PRESS LTD., Lavenham, Suffolk.

Contents

Preface

Foreword

CHAPTER I. Introduction 1

CHAPTER II. Material and Techniques 3
Recording of the cry 3
The babies studied 3
Recording situations 4
Technical data on recording sound spectrography and oscillography .. 7

CHAPTER III. Acoustic Attributes of the Cry Signals 9
1. Length 9
2. Pitch 10
3. Shift 10
4. Voice 10
5. Melody types 10
6. Continuity of signal 10
7. Glottal plosives 10
8. Vocal fry 13
9. Nasality 13
10. Tenseness 13
11. Subharmonic break 13
Limitations of the method 13
Inter-observer reliability 13

CHAPTER IV. Sound Spectrography 15
Length 15
Pitch 17
Shift 17
Voice 17

Subharmonic break 17
Melody form 17
Nasality 17
Glottal plosives 17
Vocal fry 17
Continuity of signal 17
Tenseness 19
Characteristics of the different cry types 21

CHAPTER V. Human Identification of the Cry Signals 23
Identification of the cries by observers 23
Comparison of the spectrographic and auditory identification 26
Summary of the auditory identification 29

CHAPTER VI. Studies of Cries from 'Abnormal' Babies 30
The 'Cri du chat' syndrome 30
Down's syndrome 30
'Brain damaged' children 32

CHAPTER VII. Value of Cry Studies 36
Future acoustical studies 37
Accoustical features of the cries we have studied 37
Developmental course of cries 38
Auditory identification of personal characteristics of cry 38

APPENDIX 40

REFERENCES 41

Preface

All babies cry, and it would seem surprising that so little work has been done on the nature of their cry. Everyone responsible for the care of newborn babies recognises the high pitched cry of the baby with cerebral damage, and many paediatricians are conversant with the cry of the cretin, the growling low pitched cry of the Cornelia de Lange syndrome, the feeble cry of the severely hypotonic infant, the cri du chat, the whimper of the seriously ill child, or the hoarse cry of the child with a laryngeal infection. Mothers in a newborn nursery claim to be able to recognise the cry of their own child.

Professor John Lind, Professor Olé Wasz-Höckert and their colleagues have now put all this on to a sound scientific basis by their fascinating, important and painstaking spectrographic studies of the infant's cry, and the Spastics Society and Heinemann are to be congratulated on persuading these workers to put all their experience together into this single detailed book, which will be of interest and value to so many paediatricians.

No one interested in babies can fail to find this book of tremendous interest.

R. S. Illingworth
Professor of Child Health

Foreword

Not very long ago most of the work done at maternity hospitals was solely involved with the care of the sick. Now, however, improved standards of health among today's mothers have somewhat altered the nature of this work. Among other things, increased time has been devoted to other aspects of maternity care concerning both mother and child, and we can now allow ourselves to be more concerned with psychological factors in maternity care. These developments make possible a more individual type of care for the newborn infant. The newborn is a person, and — even more important — he is a person who cannot be placed into a particular mould and cared for in a prescribed, rigid fashion. By allowing more time for the care of each child, it thus becomes possible to consider every child's individual needs, and these needs make themselves known through the medium of the cry. However, a precondition to carrying this out is that one understands what the baby is trying to say when he cries.

We are at present pursuing investigations on the baby's cry, and observing the extent to which different types of infant cry can be identified with the aid of spectrographic analyses. We have also investigated the extent to which these same types of cry can be distinguished by auditory methods. Finally, we have analysed and classified different types of cry in healthy children and statistically demonstrated the variations that occur.

It is already a common experience among paediatricians that certain sicknesses occurring in infants can bring about a definite and often readily observable change in the cry. With normal material as a basis for comparison, identification of the pathological cry becomes an even more likely possibility. The recognition of these pathological cries may eventually lead to increased possibilities in diagnosing different illnesses in their early stages.

Acknowledgements

Throughout our research we have been greatly aided by the kind help and invaluable advice of many experts. We are especially happy to acknowledge our deep appreciation to Dr. Gunnar Fant, Professor, Head of the Department of Speech Communication, Royal Institute of Technology (KTH), Stockholm; Dr. Antti Sovijärvi, Professor of Phonetics, University of Helsinki; Dr. Carl Wegelius, Professor, Director of the Wenner-Gren Research Laboratory; and Dr. Katarina Michelsson, at the time at the Children's Clinic, University of Helsinki. We also wish to express our sincere gratitude to all personnel in the above institutions and hospitals who have helped us in carrying out our studies, collecting material and working towards the solutions of the many problems we have been faced with in our work.

It would have been impossible to continue our research without economic support from the National Institute of Health, Bethesda, Maryland, the Association for the Aid of Crippled Children, New York, the Finnish Medical Research Committee, the Ane and Signe Gyllenberg Foundation, Helsinki and the Thyra Svensson's Foundation, Stockholm. We wish to thank these organizations for their essential aid.

We are grateful for the additional support which we have received from the journal *Developmental Medicine and Child Neurology*, and particularly to its editors, Dr. Ronald Mac Keith and Dr. Martin Bax.

The authors wish to thank Mr. Hilding Johansson for the demanding task of preparing the photographic material for this book.

CHAPTER I

Introduction

'Random', 'non-expressive' and 'diffuse' and similar terms have been used to describe the utterances of babies (Gesell 1940, Osgood 1953, Spitz 1963). Other writers such as Miller (1951), Sherman (1927) and van Riper (1954) suggest that the cry of a baby has little intent or meaning and that the nature of the discomfort that causes it could not be identified by the type of vocalisation. Developmentally orientated representatives of the behavioural sciences (such as Allport 1960), have approached the subject of the baby's cry from the standpoint of the well-known theory of response differentiation. They also maintain that the infant's vocalisation at birth, and for some time thereafter, is random and undifferentiated, and that it gradually becomes differentiated as a function of age.

We believed that infants' cries are meaningful, and if correctly interpreted, could convey information to the adult. This view accorded with that of Bühler (1930), Hurlock (1950), and the more phonetically orientated Trojan (1957) and Berry and Eisenson (1956), who all argue strongly for the expressive function of pre-verbal vocalisation. The study here reported describes the spectrographic analysis and identification of the cry in normal newborns and young infants during their pre-verbal state. It is supplemented by a report on auditory identification of cries by a variety of people with different amounts of experience with infants.

Normal material has been collected in certain specific and everyday situations in order to find acoustically measurable criteria to define the normal range of crying. Such criteria are essential to allow us to define a normal or abnormal cry objectively. A further application of this study will be the definition of specific acoustical criteria of abnormal cries and the correlation of them with the clinical conditions. We make some preliminary reports on these studies in Chapter VIII.

Many different aspects of crying of babies have already been studied. Illingworth (1955, 1957) has reported comprehensively on the motivations or somatic bases of vocalization in infancy. His lists include various avoidance and frustration situations.

Aldrich *et al.* (1945) and Brazelton (1962) have studied the time and quantity of crying.

Karelitz *et al.* have demonstrated tape recorded cries of normal and abnormal infants (1960), and in later studies paid special attention to their cry latencies and thresholds (1962, Fisichelli and Karelitz 1963). Several investigators (Fairbanks 1942, Lynip 1951, Ostwald *et al.* 1962, Minnigerode 1963, Ringel *et al.* 1964, Sedláčková 1964, Truby and Lind 1965, Greenberg *et al.* 1967) have studied cry parameters, especially the pitch, sound pressure, harmonic spectrum and the duration of the cry.

Electroacoustical analysis has also been used earlier in studying the effects of emotional stress on the adult human voice (Friedhoff *et al.* 1962, 1964). Sound spectrography has been used in medical research by phoneticians, laryngologists (Palva 1958,

Kyttä 1964) and cardiologists (McKusick 1958, Landtman *et al.* 1964). Some specific, acoustical qualities in the preverbal vocal communication of the normal babies have been measured adequately by sound spectrography and the situations concerned recognized by adult listeners (Wasz-Höckert *et al.* 1963, 1964a, b). Bosma *et al.* (1965a,b) have reported on normal and abnormal cries in newborn babies using sound spectrography and simultaneous cineroentgenography of their articulatory organs. Our present research group (Lind *et al.* 1965a) have shown certain specific acoustic patterns in the cry of a brain-damaged, asphyctic newborn. We have also demonstrated that several types of abnormal crying can be identified auditorily by paediatricians (Partanen *et al.* 1967).

CHAPTER II

Material and Techniques

Recording of the Cry

The cry recordings were made at the School of Midwifery of Helsinki (birth cries and one-day pain cries), at the Southern Maternity Hospital of Stockholm (1-9 day pain and hunger cries), at the Infants' Home of the Deaconess Institute of Helsinki and in private homes in Helsinki (6-215 days pain, hunger and pleasure cries). Four hundred and nineteen cry signals from 351 infants in six age groups have been analysed (Table I). The cries have been divided into four categories: birth, pain, hunger, pleasure (see page 4). Only one cry from each infant has been analysed in the different categories.

The Babies Studied

Only infants born at full term, following uneventful pregnancies and normal deliveries, to healthy mothers were accepted in the study. All of them had a 9 or 10 point score in the Apgar scale 1 and 5 minutes after birth. The birth weight varied between 2600 and 4390 g. The weight of the children was noted at the time of each recording. However, in this study we will not report correlations of the findings with weight or sex, but only with age, following negative results in pilot studies. The babies studied were all born of parents of Finnish or Swedish origin and babies born to parents who are recent immigrants were excluded. We have some evidence, however, that racial features are not significant in respect to the baby's cry signal.

All the children included in this study are considered to be completely healthy and normal. All pathological cases were carefully excluded and all the infants were examined by a paediatrician. Complete clinical data are available for all of the children, but details will not be given here.

TABLE I

Cry situation, age and sex. Italicised numbers refer to infants in whom cry analysis has been performed in more than one situation

	Age Group									
	1 0–1d	2 2–3d	3 4–5d	4 6–7d	5 8–9d	6 10–30d	7 1–3mo	8 4–5mo	9 6–7mo	Total
Birth	77 *10*									77
Pain	10	10	10	10	10	10 *10*	20 *10*	20 *10*	20 *10*	120
Hunger	10	10	10	10	10	25	25 *6*	25 *6*	25 *6*	150
Pleasure							24	24	24	72
Total cries studied	97	20	20	20	20	35	69	69	69	419
Boys	39	12	6	11	10	8	29	18	32	165
Girls	48	8	14	9	10	17	24	35	21	186
Infants	87	20	20	20	20	25	53	53	53	351

Recording Situations

The problem was to select cry signals for study which might be expected to be specific signals. It is clearly not possible for an adult to know what a particular baby 'feels' at a given time, and we decided to use easily definable situations as constants in order to facilitate the collection of a sampling of cries, which we shall call *situational cries*. There are difficulties in such selection, but we believe the signal types chosen are ones which clinically can be identified clearly from other parameters, not merely from their purely auditory qualities. With the exception of the birth cry, babies whom the nurses reported cried a lot were not studied, as it was difficult to be certain that we knew the reason for their crying at any particular time. In all babies we have studied, the reason for their crying at any particular time appeared clear cut.

In describing the situations one is faced with the problem of deciding what language one should use to describe the baby's state. Is it permissible to speak of the baby being 'happy' or 'angry'? In our opinion, the baby's total situation can only be explained from the adult's view and therefore we have not been afraid to use adult terms to describe the baby's behavioural state.

The four situations in which we have made recordings are as follows.

1. *The birth cry* (Fig. 1). The recorder attended the delivery standing beside the midwife with his microphone. This he held to the baby's mouth as soon as the head had been delivered. Sometimes a cry was recorded before the rest of the body had been delivered. The normal sequence of events is that the baby takes one or two gasping inspirations and then gives a cry. This is the cry we have recorded and studied. Sometimes before a clear signal is heard the baby's mouth will have been cleaned and the airway cleared by gentle suction. The signal we are studying was always obtained within the first five minutes after the head was delivered. The recording was always completed before the cord was clamped.

The birth cries were all recorded in the same delivery room (in Helsinki). In any modern maternity unit the level of ambient noise is very high and to eliminate this it was clearly necessary to use a microphone with a small recording field. The microphone had to be held within 1″ to 1½″ of the baby's mouth. After pilot studies the midwives became very interested in the project and tried to deliver the baby in such a way that the recorder's job was made easy.

2. *The pain cries* (Fig. 2) were recorded when the baby was having the BCG or PDT (triple) vaccination or simply after pinching the skin over the infant's biceps. In future studies we plan to use a more standardised stimulus (a prick from a modified Heaf gun) but we do not believe this will alter our results. These recordings were made 5-30 minutes after the meal when the infants were dry, calm and comfortable, but fully awake in their cots or in the arms of the nurse. The babies were in the state described by Prechtl (1964) as State 3. It would clearly have been wrong to use painful stimuli when the baby was in State 1 as the cry might then be interpreted as one of irritation at being woken up. The cry signal during the first vocalized expiratory cycle after the pain stimulus has been selected for the study. Additionally, the interval between the stimulus and the beginning of the cry reaction and the interval between the first and second

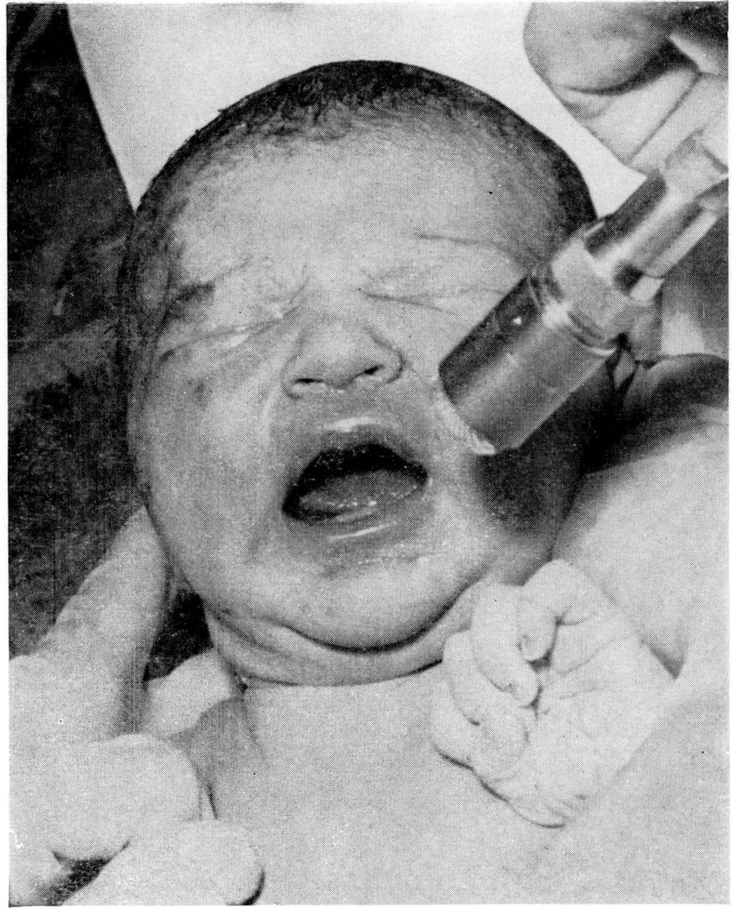

Fig. 1. The birth cry

vocalized respiration, as well as the total length of the cry period after the stimulus, have been measured. These results have been reported elsewhere (Lind *et al.* 1966).

3. *The hunger cry* (Fig. 3) has been recorded at 4 hours $\pm$ 20 min. after the previous meal when the infant is crying steadily and all the motives for his discomfort, other than hunger, have been excluded as far as possible. The intake of food at the previous feed must have been average and the behaviour in the intervening period not remarkable.

Even so, it is not, of course, possible to be certain that the cry is given entirely because of hunger. It might be that the baby wanted handling. However, the eagerness with which the baby accepted the bottle or the breast after the recording made us feel certain that our explanation of the cause of the cry was the right one. Each recording was about 5 minutes in duration, and from this the signal to be analysed has been selected. Although hunger cries were collected as early as 12 hours, it is difficult at this time to be certain that the situation truly represents hunger. Relatively few cries therefore have been collected in the first three days of life.

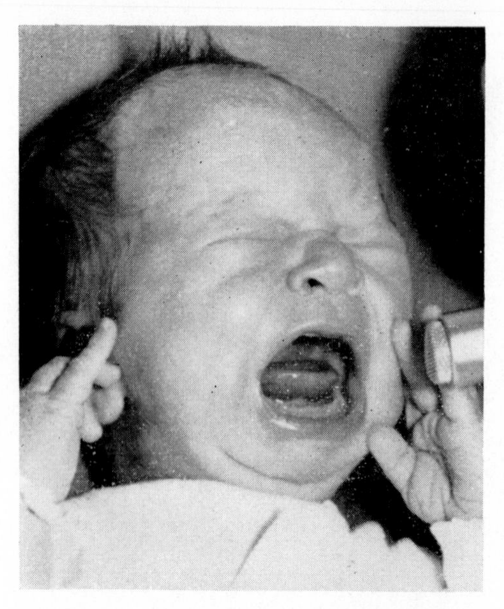

Fig. 2. Baby giving a pain cry. Our impression is that during the pain cry there is marked tension in the circum-aural muscle channel, the eyes are often screwed up and the baby frowns. With the first cry the arms are often flexed, the fists clenched. Compare with Figure 3.

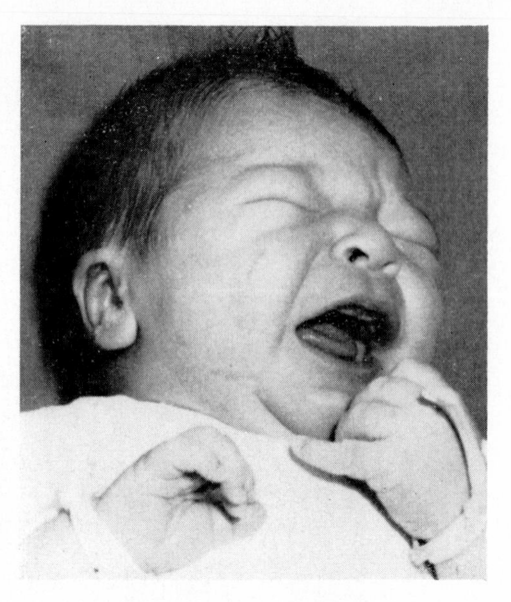

Fig. 3. Hunger cry. Here the baby's face is less tense. The posture of the arms is unremarkable.

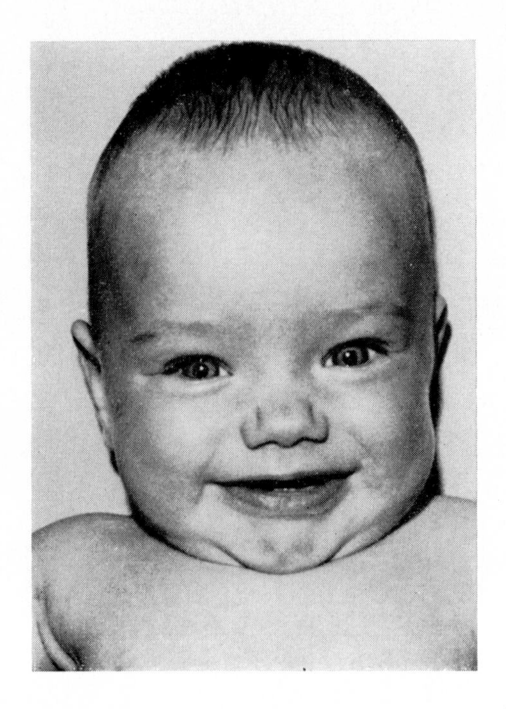

Fig. 4. The pleasure cry.

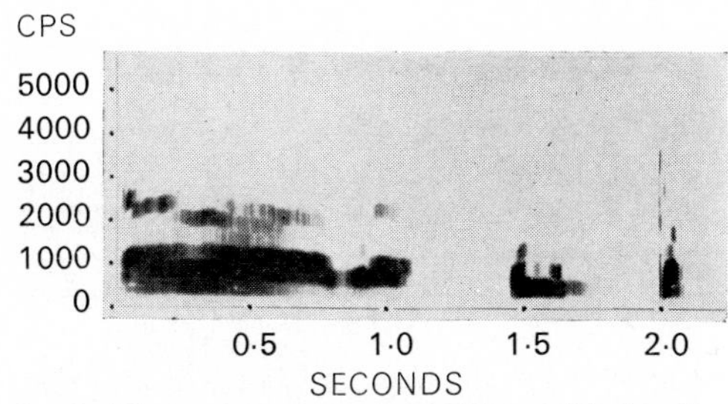

Fig. 5. Pleasure cry recorded with a wide band filter. (In spectrograms throughout the book, pitch is recorded in cycles per second on the vertical axis, and time in seconds on the horizontal axis. The scale is 1 inch to 1 second throughout.)

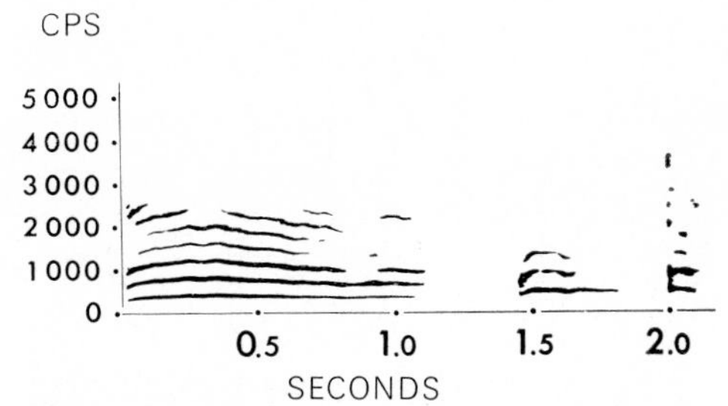

Fig. 6. The same cry as in Fig. 5 recorded with a narrow band filter.

4. *The pleasure signals* (Fig. 4) have been recorded in a situation where the infant, having been fed and changed, was lying comfortably on the bed or in the arms of the mother or the nurse. This is the first sound the baby makes that can be readily identified and associated with a specific pleasure situation; it does not arise till around 3 months. The baby is usually looking at the adult who may be stimulating him with gentle movements or making soft noises. The baby frequently smiles at the adult and gives every sign of being content. The duration of each recording was about 5 minutes.

With regard to the long-lasting *hunger* and *pleasure* cries, we have encountered some difficulty in deciding which part of the recording should be used for analysis. These samples have been chosen by the phonetician, who alone decided which specific cries were to be analysed. It was not possible to make a detailed analysis of the 5 minutes, but the cry samples selected by him were checked for accuracy of length by comparing them with the lengths of all the cry signals, including those not selected for the study. No significant differences were found. The samples analysed were therefore typical examples of the whole.

Technical Data on Recording Sound Spectrography and Oscillography

In making the cry recordings, two high quality tape recorders have been used; Movicorder Stereo A Two* and Nagra III**. The last one is a battery-driven and easily portable recorder. It is more convenient to employ in clinical situations since it can easily be brought close to the infant, thus avoiding unnecessary movement of the baby.

A tape speed of 7½ in./sec. was found to be adequate for recording quality and tape editing. A pressure gradient dynamic microphone AKG D 58***, supplied with a windscreen, was used. The microphone was placed horizontally towards one of the corners of the mouth, at a distance of 1–1½ in. This microphone, although having a very small recording field, still has a satisfactory frequency response in the range of 100 — 8000 c/s and considerably reduces noise and echo. As most of the components of the cry are in the 100 to 5000 c/s range this microphone is quite adequate.

* Made by Movic Co. Copenhagen.
**Model NPH, made by Kudelski, Lausanne.
***Made by AKG, Vienna.

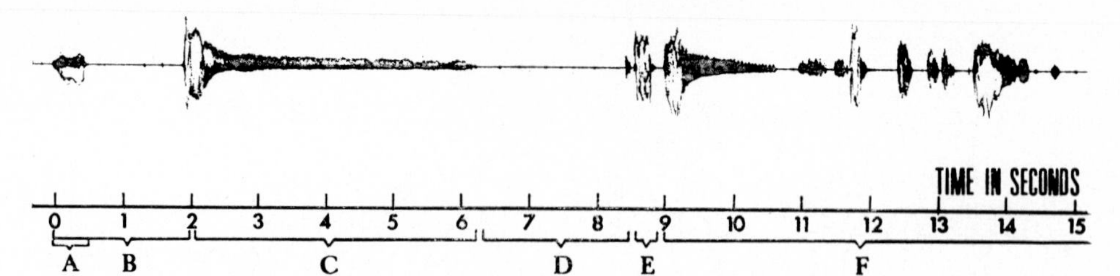

Fig. 7. Oscillogram of a pain cry. (A) the baby is pinched and the examiner says the word 'now'; (B) represents the first latency period; (C) is the first expiratory cry; (D) is the second latency period; (E) a phonated inspiration; (F) second cry signals and phonated inspirations; (G) the signals gradually get smaller and smaller. The cry signal (C) is the one which we invariably analyse.

For the spectrographic analysis we have used the *Sona-Graph* model 661-A (Kay Electric Co. New Jersey) and *Voiceprint* (Voiceprint Laboratories, Inc. New Jersey). For details of the technique, see e.g. Potter *et al.* (1947), Wasz-Höckert *et al.* (1962, 1963). These two spectrum analyzers both have a wide band filter (300 c/s) and a narrow band filter (45 c/s); for our purposes of measuring the fundamental frequency (pitch) we found the narrow band filter the most adequate (see Figs. 5 and 6). In this study we have not attempted to find speech sound characteristics (vowels and consonants) in the cry, as Irwin *et al.* (1952) attempted to do.

For the length measurements we have used a direct indicating amplitude recorder, the *Mingograph* (Elema Schönander, Solna, Sweden), see Fig. 7.

At the end of this book there is a record which gives examples of the cries we shall be describing. For analytical studies records are not satisfactory and taped recordings are used.*

*Those wishing to work in the field may wish to consult original tapes and these are available from the authors.

CHAPTER III

Acoustic Attributes of the Cry Signals

A cry signal (Joppich 1964, Lanyon *et al.* 1960) consists of the total vocalisation occurring during a single expiration or inspiration. True inspiratory cries are rare in normal infants and most noises that one hears are mechanical in origin, i.e. they are due to some obstruction of the airway and not to an intentional vocalisation initiated from the central nervous system.

In order to describe and analyse such signals we have selected several terms and methods used by Jakobson *et al.* (1952) for studying opposing sound qualities, or distinctive features and applied them in the differential analysis of infant cries. Following pilot studies 10 phonetic items were selected for use in analysis. Some of these items have been retained, not for use in distinguishing normal cries but because of preliminary indications that they will be significant in pathological conditions.

Distinctive features which have been classified consist of the following: (1) 5 melody types (rising-falling, falling, flat, rising, falling-rising); (2) continuity of sound; (3) voiced vs. voiceless signals; (4) oral vs. nasal signals; (5) lax vs. tense signals. Length and pitch have been measured. Other phenomena occurring in the cry signals have been analysed: the occurrence of glottal plosives, vocal fry and subharmonic break*.

These acoustic attributes have been analysed according to the following criteria.

1. Length

At first sight the length might be thought the easiest part of the cry signal to analyse objectively. It might be desirable to measure all the phonation during any expiration but this would make analysis so time-consuming as to be impossible. Measuring the time between the first and last vocalisations during a single expiration does not prove a useful rule in practice. For example, with the hunger cry it is common to have a series of plosives with widely varying latent periods between them. These are followed by a more sustained signal. It was found that if the plosive were included in the length measurements, the length of signals varied very widely and only if the main signal alone was included did more consistent figures emerge.

The same proved to be true for plosives occurring after the main cry. It was rare to find a plosive occurring in the middle of the longer sound, but where this did occur it seemed wiser to regard this as an interruption of the signal only and to include it in the measurement. Other considerations arose with the other cry signals and following much practical study with records, the length of signal was defined as the time between the first and last vocalisations of more than 0·4 sec. This was irrespective of the size of the latency period between the signals or the occurrence of any shorter signals between the longer one of 0·4 sec. While the rule may sound clumsy, it is easy to apply, as will emerge during the study. The exception to this occurs when there are

*These phonetic terms are defined on pages 10-13.

plosives only (Fig. 17). This happens only in hunger cries and in this the time between the first and last vocalisation is measured.

It is not possible to make measurements of greater accuracy than 0·1 sec. as, although amplification for making the spectrograms is standard, the print-out rate varies by about 0·1 sec. when the vocalisation begins or ends with a minimal sound pressure. Pilot studies show that such errors can arise (Fig. 8).

2. Pitch

(a) *Minimum pitch:* The lowest measured voiced point of the cry. No attention has been paid to the vocal fry.

(b) *General pitch:* The pitch level that dominates the cry. When the level is evidently very unstable, this measurement has not been made.

(c) *Maximum pitch:* The highest measured voiced point of the cry. The shift is measured separately. If the maximum pitch is the same as the general pitch it is not measured. All the pitch measurements have been made with the accuracy of 10 c/s. When voicelessness increases to a certain level, the pitch cannot be measured.

3. Shift

The occurrence of shift has been recorded and a cry classified as with or without shift. The shift is a sudden upward or downward change in pitch level somewhat similar to what occurs in yodelling, but the pitch changes in infant cries are irregular. In Figure 8 there is an illustration of a cry with shift. The new pitch established by the shift can be measured, and this has been done.

4. Voice

Three different gradings have been made from the spectrograms: voiced, half-voiced and voiceless. In Figure 8 there is a voiced cry; in Figure 9, a voiceless one and in Figure 10 a half-voiced cry.

5. Melody Types

The different melody types have been defined as a change in the pitch level, when exceeding 10 per cent of the pitch during more than 10 per cent of the length of the cry. Examples of typical melody types are: Figure 11—a rising-falling type of melody, Figure 12—falling pain cry, Figure 13—rising pleasure signal, Figure 14—flat pleasure signal, Figures 9, 16 — no melody form (when the cry is (1) totally voiceless, (2) contains only glottal plosives or shorter sounds that are less than 0·4 sec.).

6. Continuity of Signal

Any signal containing two or more vocalisations of 0·4 sec. or more in length is classified as an interrupted signal (Fig. 16).

7. Glottal Plosives

The cries have been divided into three groups: those in which glottal plosives occur in the same cry signal with other types of vocalisation, those which are only glottal plosives and those with no glottal plosives.

It is only in pleasure cries that the baby begins to produce labial or palatal plosives. In order to distinguish different types of plosives, wide band analysis is required, but in this study all plosives are classed as glottal plosives (Fig. 17).

CPS
5000
4000
3000
2000
1000
0
0.5
1.0
1.5
2.0
2.5
3.0
SECONDS

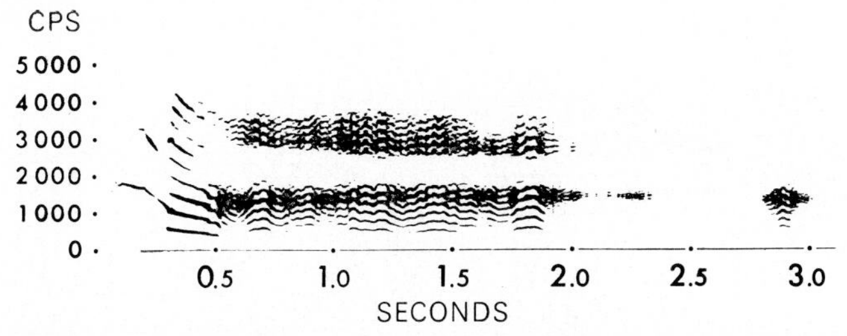

Fig. 8. This demonstrates the difficulties in measurements. When the cry signal (a pain cry) begins and ends with minimal sound pressure it is difficult to decide where the signal begins and ends.

The pitch is minimal at about one second when the distance between the harmonics is at its lowest. It is difficult to decide on the general pitch of this cry. Here it would not be measured. The maximum pitch occurs at ·3 seconds. The cry also demonstrates shift well in the period ·1 to ·3 seconds and there is a clear change in the overall pitch. The fundamental at the beginning of the cry is about 2000, which is the pitch of the shift.

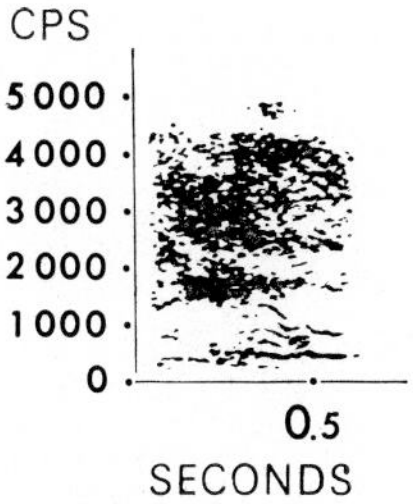

CPS
5000
4000
3000
2000
1000
0
0.5
SECONDS

Fig. 9. A voiceless birth cry.

CPS
5000
4000
3000
2000
1000
0
0.5
1.0
1.5
SECONDS

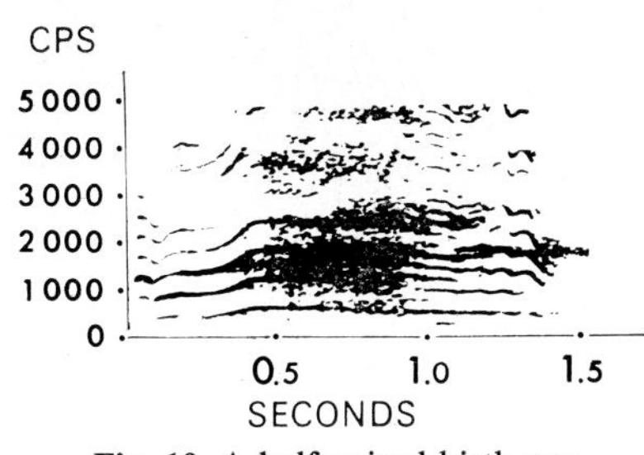

Fig. 10. A half-voiced birth cry.

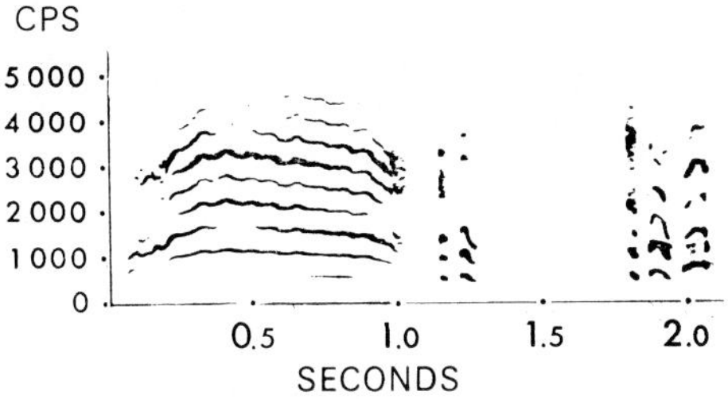

CPS
5000
4000
3000
2000
1000
0
0.5
1.0
1.5
2.0
SECONDS

Fig. 11. A rising-falling melody in a hunger cry. Note also the glottal plosives.

CPS
5000
4000
3000
2000
1000
0
0.5
1.0
1.5
2.0
2.5
3.0
3.5
4.0
4.5
SECONDS

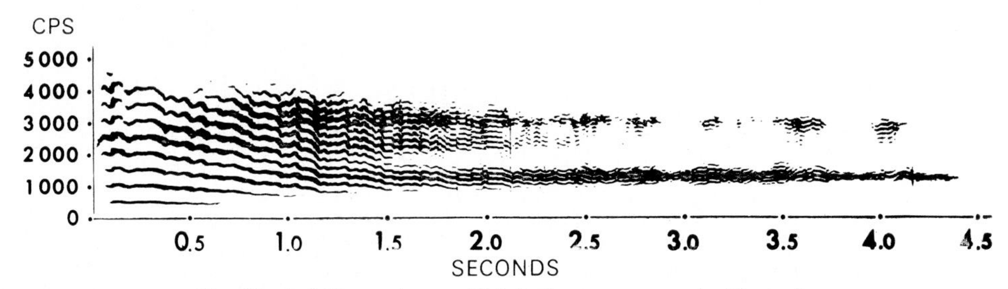

Fig. 12. A falling pain cry. This is the same cry as in Figure 7.

CPS
5000
4000
3000
2000
1000
0
0.5
1.0
SECONDS

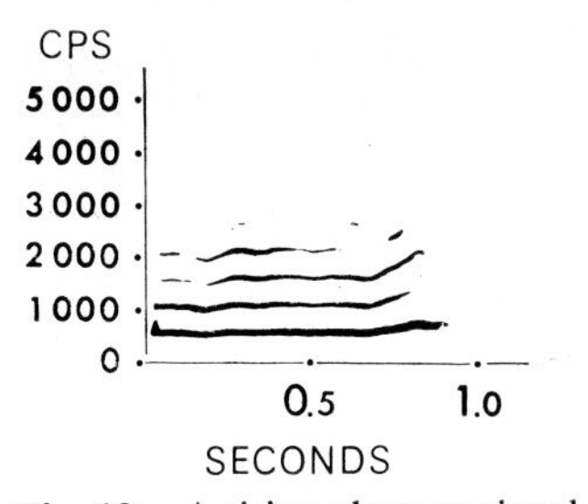

Fig. 13. A rising pleasure signal.

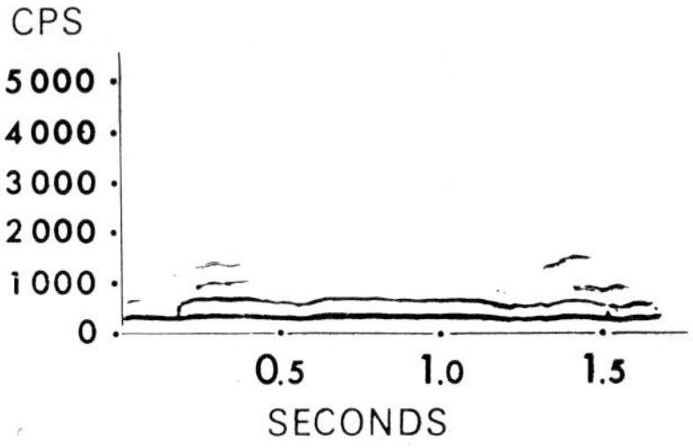

CPS
5000
4000
3000
2000
1000
0
0.5
1.0
1.5
SECONDS

Fig. 14. A flat pleasure signal. This cry also demonstrates nasality.

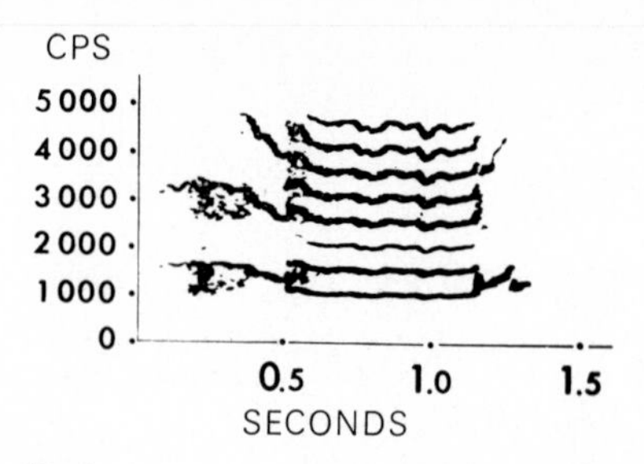

Fig. 15. A rare cry, a pain cry with a falling-rising pattern.

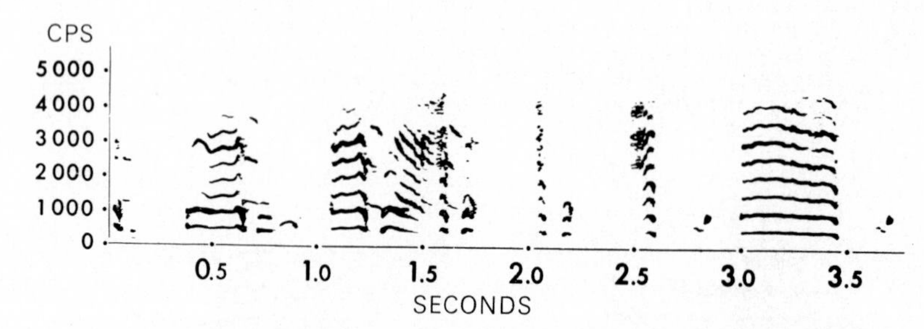

Fig. 16. An interrupted signal (a pain cry) with many vocalisations more than ·4 of a second.

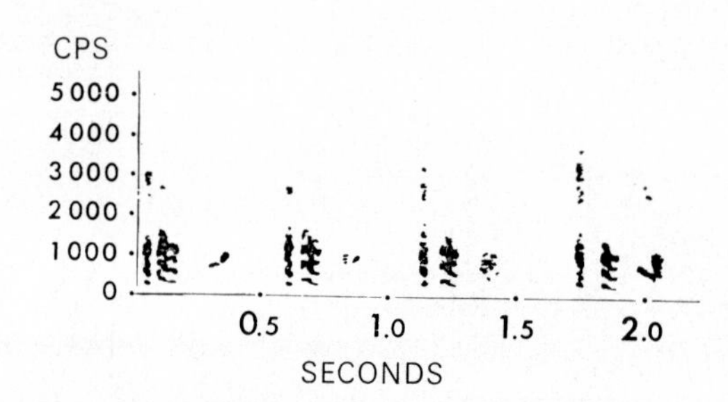

Fig. 17. A hunger cry of only glottal plosives.

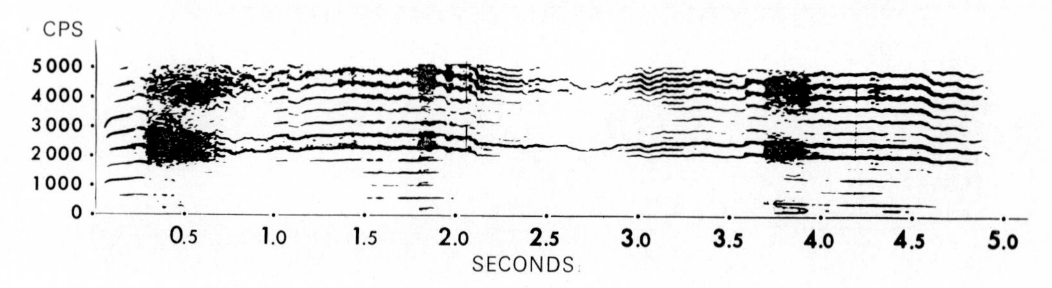

Fig. 18. A tense pain cry with tense upper harmonics. Note the voiceless sections around ·5 seconds and 3·8 seconds. This cry also demonstrates subharmonic break, which can be seen most clearly from about 2·1 seconds to 3·3 seconds, although traces of it can be seen right through to the end of the cry.

8. Vocal Fry

Vocal fry, or 'glottal roll' or creak, is an unperiodical phonation of the vocal folds in a lower frequency range, that is below the normal pitch register. It appears in infants' cries as in adult speech, quite often at the end of a phonation, falling in pitch and intensity. The vocal fry is seen in the spectrograms as trembling, narrow harmonics of a low intensity. In analysing the material, a division has been made between cries with more than 0·2 sec. of vocal fry and those with less or no vocal fry. In the falling pattern, seen in Fig. 12, there is vocal fry at the end of the cry at 3·0 sec., at 3·4 sec., and from 3·7 sec. to 4·0 sec.

9. Nasality

Nasality occurs in infant's vocalisation most commonly during the partial or total closing of the oral cavities and the opening of the nasal cavity. A rough grouping has been made of cries with and without nasality. The nasal voice is poor in intensity and only the first harmonics are amplified. A nasal cry is illustrated in Figure 14.

10. Tenseness

A tense voice is strained and strident. Here again, only two types of signals have been distinguished: tense and lax. Tenseness increases the intensity of the upper harmonics and that of the range of fricative noise in voiceless cries (see Fig. 18). A good example of a lax cry is present in Figure 11.

11. Subharmonic Break

We have used the term 'subharmonic break' to designate a complex cry signal, composed of the normal spectrum of a fundamental with its harmonics and another simultaneous series of harmonics lasting for more than 0·2 sec. The physiology of this phenomenon will not be discussed in this study (see Fig. 18).

Limitations of the Method

Because of the sound spectrographic method used, it is not possible to measure voice, vocal fry, nasality, tenseness and subharmonic break quantitatively, as for example with length and pitch. Therefore, in rating these we have to rely solely upon the evaluation of the investigator. The investigator naturally benefited from his knowledge of the sounds, but, as will be shown overleaf, despite the qualitative nature of the description it is possible to demonstrate good inter-observer reliability.

Inter-observer Reliability

The reliability of the ratings performed by the investigator was determined by a random sampling of 40 spectrograms which were used in this study; they were evaluated by a group of 6 'judges', who were all employed as sound technicians at the Finnish Radio Corporation. Each judge was required to rate the 40 spectrograms with respect to the following attributes which were felt to be the most subjective items in the analysis:

(1) Voice (voiced — half-voiced — voiceless)
(2) Vocal fry (+ —)
(3) Nasality (+ —)
(4) Tenseness (+ —)
(5) Subharmonic break (+ —).

Before making the ratings the observers were given instructions very similar to the rating criteria given on the preceding pages.

The ratings of each judge were cross-tabulated against the ratings of the investigator. The number of concordant ratings were counted for each judge separately and divided by the total number of rated spectrograms (Table II).

TABLE II

Proportions of concordant ratings between 6 judges and the phonetician

Judge	1	2	3	4	5	6	Mean 1-6
Voice I*	0·62	0·45	0·82	0·75	0·78	0·78	0·70
Voice II**	0·72	0·80	0·85	0·88	0·92	0·85	0·84
Vocal fry	0·80	0·65	0·95	0·90	0·75	0·88	0·82
Nasality	0·90	0·62	0·92	0·72	0·82	0·90	0·81
Tenseness	0·95	0·92	0·95	0·85	0·95	0·95	0·93
Subharmonic break	0·98	0·82	0·95	0·98	0·90	0·92	0·93

*three-category rating.
**dichotomous: voiced and half-voiced combined into one class.

The rating of the voice in three grades is naturally less reliable than rating in only two. The overall concordance rises from 0·70 (three-grade case) to 0·84 (two-grade case). Some variation is present in the trichotomous ratings of the judges (notice especially the low level of concordance of one of the judges). In the vocal fry and nasality attributes, the overall reliability is a little more than 0·80. Among the five attributes, tenseness and subharmonic break are easiest to recognize. Both have an overall reliability of 0·93. This cross checking experiment indicates that an experienced investigator has the ability to determine and rate the mentioned attributes in a reliable way and that others can be trained to make identical assessments.

CHAPTER IV

Sound Spectrography

In the following, the four signal types (birth, pain, hunger, pleasure) are compared using the spectrographic and acoustical attributes described earlier. The signals are divided into two groups according to the age* of the infant: 0-1 and 1-7 months. The attributes will be analysed first separately, then in a simultaneous multivariate manner. The univariate analysis reveals group differences in the several attributes between the signal classes; the multivariate analysis results in classification rules for separate signals.

The univariate differences between the signal classes are tested using X^2, F, unit normal deviate, and hypergeometric distributions as well as the Wilcoxon test, according to the statistical requirements of the testing situation. The respective risk probabilities are indicated with $p(X^2)$, p(F), p(z), p(H), and p(W). If any of these exceeds ·05, it is considered not significant and will not be presented. Numbers of signals in the different signal classes have been given earlier.

The purposes of the multivariate analysis of the present data are (1) to screen out the relatively independent combination of attributes (i.e. those that represent different common and specific factors), and (2) to predict a separate signal's type using these attributes simultaneously. To accomplish this, the data were subjected to factor analysis and robot data screening (Sterling and Pollack 1965). The function of factor analysis is reducing the attribute space to be used in the prediction by removing redundant attributes. In the analysis, principal axis solution was applied with Varimax rotation. Two analyses were carried out: one for the age group 0-1 months, the other for the 1-7 months group. Eight principal axes were extracted in both analyses before rotation. The variables submitted to the analyses are those listed earlier.

Computer data screening selects the attribute subset that discriminates best between the signal classes. The routine starts with the predicted attribute (signal class) and adds predictor attributes one by one on the basis of the improvement in joint predictability provided by the successive sets of predictor attributes. It results in classification rules of the following form: 'given a signal with position 'a' in attribute x_1, position 'b' in attribute x_2, and position 'c' in attribute x_3, it belongs to the signal class y_1, this rule can be expected correct in p per cent of the future cases.' In this application, predictors were searched for until no significant error reduction took place. All the attributes used were classified into 2 or 3 classes.

Length (Table III)

There are marked differences between the relatively long pain signals and the rest of the signals. Birth, hunger, and pleasure signals are rather similar in length.

*Age does not seem to have much effect on the characteristics of the signals. Accordingly, the data have been pooled into just two age classes.

TABLE III

Mean length (sec.) in signal classes

	Birth	*Pain*	*Hunger*	*Pleasure*
0-1 *month*				
Mean	1·1	2·6	1·3	
s.d.	·4	1·5	·6	
Overall p(F) < ·001				
Birth vs. pain: p(z) < ·001				
Birth vs. hunger: p(z) < ·05				
Pain vs. hunger: p(z) < ·001				
1-7 *months*				
Mean		2·7	1·2	1·1
s.d.		1·1	·6	·5
Overall p(F) < ·001				
Pain vs. hunger < ·001				
Pain vs. pleasure < ·001				

A procedure for making comparisons between groups within the subsets selected — fixing the overall significance level — might have been more desirable (see for example Gabriel 1964, 1966) but it was felt this pairwise analysis was adequate provided it was cautiously interpreted.

TABLE V

Occurrence and pitch of shift in signal classes

	Birth	*Pain*	*Hunger*	*Pleasure*
0-1 *month*				
Proportion with shift	·18	·32	·04	
Overall p(χ^2) < ·01				
Birth vs. hunger: p(χ^2) < ·05				
Pain vs. hunger: p(χ^2) < ·001				
Pitch of shift, cps Median	870	1140	*	
Birth vs. pain: p(W) < ·05				
1-7 *months*				
Proportion with shift		·38	—	·19
Pain vs. hunger: p(H) < ·001				
Pain vs. pleasure: p(χ^2) < ·001				
Hunger vs. pleasure: p(H) < ·01				

*not calculated

TABLE IV

Mean pitch (cps.) in signal classes

	Birth	*Pain*	*Hunger*	*Pleasure*
0-1 *month*				
General pitch:				
Mean	500	530	470	
s.d.	60	80	40	
Max. pitch:				
Mean	550	650	550	
s.d.	70	100	60	
Min. pitch:				
Mean	450	410	390	
s.d.	60	90	60	
Overall p(F) < ·001 (gen, max., min.)				
Birth vs. pain: p(z) < ·05 (gen.)				
p(z) < ·001 (max.)				
p(z) < ·01 (min.)				
Birth vs. hunger: p(z) < ·001 (gen., min.)				
Pain vs. hunger: p(z) < ·001 (gen., max.)				
1-7 *months*				
General pitch:				
Mean		530	500	440
s.d.		80	70	90
Max. pitch:				
Mean		680	520	650
s.d.		80	80	200
Min. pitch:				
Mean		380	420	360
s.d.		70	70	140
Overall p(F) < ·001 (gen., max.)				
p(F) < ·05 (min.)				
Pain vs. hunger: p(z) < ·05 (gen.)				
p(z) < ·001 (max.)				
p(z) < ·01 (min.)				
Pain vs. pleasure: p(z) < ·001 (gen.)				
Hunger vs. pleasure: p(z) < ·001 (gen., max.)				
p(z) < ·01 (min.)				

Pitch (Table IV)

In the pitch measurements, highly significant differences between signal classes are observed mostly in general and maximum pitch (Table IV). Pain signals are the highest except in minimum pitch which reaches its highest average of 450 cps. in the birth signals. Pleasure signals are relatively low-pitched in general and minimum pitch but rather high (average 650 cps.) in maximum pitch. This is a sign of the inner variability in the pleasure signal.

Shift (Table V)

Shift occurs most in pain signals (in 30 to 40% of them, Table V). The differences in occurrence of shift between the signal classes are mostly significant. In the younger age group, there is an almost significant difference in average pitch of shift between pain (median 1140 cps.) and birth (870 cps.) signals. In the older age group, the median pitch of shift does not differ significantly between pain and pleasure signals.

Voice (Table VI)

Voice quality discriminates best between birth and other signals (Table VI). Birth signals are frequently voiceless, in contrast to the more voiced pain and hunger signals. In the older age group, no significant differences are found between the signal types, as practically all cries are voiced.

Subharmonic Break (Table VII)

Subharmonic break (Table VII) occurs most frequently in pain signals. In birth and hunger signals it occurs rather seldom. About one in five of the pleasure signals has this phenomenon.

Melody Form (Table VIII)

The signal groups are rather different in their typical melody form. Birth signals are mostly flat (·36 of them), or falling (·31), pain signals falling (·62, ·77), hunger signals rising-falling (·78 and ·81), and pleasure signals either flat (·46) or rising-falling (·31).

Nasality (Table IX)

Nasality is present mostly in the pleasure signals (·57).

Glottal Plosives (Table X)

Glottal plosives are characteristic of 50-70 per cent of hunger signals, 30-50 per cent of pain signals and less in birth and pleasure signals. Some hunger vocalizations contain only glottal plosives.

Vocal Fry (Table XI)

Most pain signals contain vocal fry, whereas it is relatively rare in the other signal types, especially in birth cries.

Continuity of Signal (Table XII)

Proportions of continuous signals are high in every signal class. Some statistically significant differences are present. This is due to the very high proportion of continuousness in birth (·94) and pleasure (1·00) signals.

TABLE VI

Voice quality in signal classes (proportions)

	Birth	*Pain*	*Hunger*
0-1 *month*			
Voiceless	·60	·07	·20
Half voiced	·35	·28	·20
Voiced	·05	·65	·60

Overall p(χ^2) < ·001
Birth vs. pain: p(χ^2) < ·001
Birth vs. hunger: p(χ^2) < ·001
Pain vs. hunger: p(χ^2) < ·05

TABLE VII

Proportion of signals with subharmonic break in signal classes

	Birth	*Pain*	*Hunger*	*Pleasure*
0-1 *month*				
Proportion	·03	·48	·10	

Overall p(χ^2) < ·001
Birth vs. pain: p(χ^2) < ·001
Pain vs. hunger: p(χ^2) < ·001

	Birth	*Pain*	*Hunger*	*Pleasure*
1-7 *months*				
Proportion		·62	·03	·22

Overall p(χ^2) < ·001
Pain vs. hunger: p(χ^2) < ·001
Pain vs. pleasure: p(χ^2) < ·001
Hunger vs. pleasure: p(χ^2) < ·001

TABLE IX

Proportion of nasal signals in signal classes

	Birth	*Pain*	*Hunger*	*Pleasure*
0-1 *month*				
Proportion	·05	·18	·11	

Overall p(χ^2) < ·05
Birth vs. pain: p(χ^2) < ·05

	Birth	*Pain*	*Hunger*	*Pleasure*
1-7 *months*				
Proportion		·25	—	·57

Overall p(χ^2) < ·001
Pain vs. hunger: p(H) < ·001
Pain vs. pleasure: p(χ^2) < ·001
Pain vs. pleasure p(χ^2) < ·001
Hunger vs. pleasure: p(H) < ·001

TABLE VIII

Melody form in signal classes (proportions)

(All the p values are based on the dichotomized attribute: rising-falling vs. other forms)

	Birth	*Pain*	*Hunger*	*Pleasure*
0-1 *month*				
Rising-falling	·13	·23	·78	
Falling	·31	·62	·01	
Rising	·03	·08	—	
Flat	·36	·02	·11	
Falling-rising	—	—	—	
No form	·16	·05	·09	

Overall p(χ^2) < ·001
Birth vs. hunger: p(χ^2) < ·001
Pain vs. hunger: p(χ^2) < ·001

	Birth	*Pain*	*Hunger*	*Pleasure*
1-7 *months*				
Rising-falling		·18	·81	·31
Falling		·77	·04	·10
Rising		·02	—	·08
Flat		·03	·01	·46
Falling-rising		—	—	·06
No form		—	·14	—

Overall p(χ^2) < ·001
Pain vs. hunger: p(χ^2) < ·001
Hunger vs. pleasure: p(χ^2) < ·001

TABLE X

Occurrence of glottal plosives in signal classes (proportions)

(All the p values based on dichotomized attribute)

	Birth	*Pain*	*Hunger*	*Pleasure*
0-1 *month*				
No glottal plosives	·79	·50	·50	
Glottal plosives	·21	·50	·37	
Only glottal plosives	—	—	·13	

Overall p(χ^2) < ·001
Birth vs. pain: p(χ^2) < ·001
Birth vs. hunger: p(χ^2) < ·001

	Birth	*Pain*	*Hunger*	*Pleasure*
1-7 *months*				
No glottal plosives		·72	·31	·90
Glottal plosives		·28	·54	·10
Only glottal plosives		—	·15	—

Overall p(χ^2) < ·001
Pain vs. hunger: p(χ^2) < ·001
Pain vs. pleasure: ‘(χ^2) < ·05
Hunger vs. pleasure: p(χ^2) < ·001

TABLE XI

Occurrence of vocal fry in signal classes

	Birth	*Pain*	*Hunger*	*Pleasure*
0-1 *month*				
Proportion	·04	·63	·28	
Overall p(χ^2) < ·001 Birth vs. pain: p(χ^2) < ·001 Birth vs. hunger: p(χ^2) < ·001 Pain vs. hunger: p(χ^2) < ·001				
1-7 *months*				
Proportion		·73	·20	·26
Overall p(X^2) < ·001 Pain vs. hunger: p(χ^2) < ·001 Pain vs. pleasure: p(χ^2) < ·001				

TABLE XII

Proportion of continuous signals in signal classes

	Birth	*Pain*	*Hunger*	*Pleasure*
0-1 *month*				
Proportion	·94	·70	·82	
Overall p(χ^2) < ·01 Birth vs. pain: p(χ^2) < ·001				
1-7 *months*				
Proportion		·73	·73	1·00
Overall p(χ^2) < ·001 Pain vs. pleasure: p(H) < ·001 Hunger vs. pleasure: p(H) < ·001				

TABLE XIII

Proportion of tense signals in signal classes

	Birth	*Pain*	*Hunger*	*Pleasure*
0-1 *month*				
Proportion	·94	·90	·42	
Overall p(χ^2) < ·001 Birth vs. hunger: p(χ^2) < ·001 Pain vs. hunger: p(χ^2) < ·001				
1-7 *months*				
Proportion		·87	·42	
Overall p(χ^2) < ·001 Pain vs. hunger: p(χ^2) < ·001 Pain vs. pleasure: p(H) < ·001 Hunger vs. pleasure: p(H) < ·001				

TABLE XIV

Cross-tabulation of melody form and length of signal

(Age group 0—1 months; absolute frequencies)

Melody form	*Length, sec.*	*Birth*	*Pain*	*Hunger*
Rising-	—1·5	8	5	46
falling	1·6—	2	9	12
Other	—1·5	53	8	9
	1·6—	14	38	7

Tenseness (Table XIII)

Birth and pain signals are very often tense; pleasure signals in this sample never. Hunger signals are intermediate (·42 of them tense).

In the age group 0-1 months, factor analysis reveals four common factors after rotation. Interpretation of them is not attempted since the interest is variable reduction only. In screening out the attributes for further analysis, the highest loading attribute (in the absolute value sense) was selected in every factor, plus those attributes that did not have any loading exceeding ·50. The first group of attributes represent common factors (having relatively high communalities), the second group specific factors (having relatively low communalities). The list of attributes adopted to the computer data screening is thus as follows:

Representing common factors:

General pitch
Flat melody form
Rising-falling melody form
Continuousness

Representing specific factors:

Length
Shift
Subharmonic break
Rising melody form
No melody form
Nasality
Glottal plosives
Lax-tense

The computer data screening showed that rising-falling melody form and length give the best prediction of an individual signal's class. Adding more attributes does not improve the predictability significantly. Table XIV is a cross-tabulation of signal type and the two best discriminating attributes. The resulting classification rules are:

(1) A signal with rising-falling melody form should be classified as a hunger signal,

(2) A signal with some other melody form (mostly flat or falling) *and* length equal or less than 1·5 sec. should be classified as a birth signal.

(3) A signal *without* a rising-falling melody form (mostly falling) *and with* length more than 1·5 sec. should be classified as a pain signal.

This rule can be expected to be correct in 71 out of a hundred classifications.

In the older age group, factor analysis resulted in the following selection of attributes:

Representing common factors:

Flat melody form
Falling melody form
General pitch

Representing specific factors:

Shift
Voice quality
Rising melody form
No melody form
Nasality
Vocal fry

These attributes were subjected to computer data screening. Three attributes were screened out as the best predictor set (Table XV). The classification rule is then:

(1) A signal with falling melody form should be classified as a pain signal,

(2) A signal with some other melody form *and* nasality *and* shift should also be classified as a pain signal,

(3) A signal with a melody form other than falling (mostly flat), *with* nasality, but *no* shift should be classified as a pleasure signal,

TABLE XV

Cross-tabulation of melody form, nasality, and shift

(Age group 1—7 months; absolute frequencies)

Melody form	*Nasality*	*Shift*	*Pain*	*Hunger*	*Pleasure*
Falling	Yes	Yes	7	—	1
		No	4	—	1
	No	Yes	11	—	2
		No	24	3	3
Other	Yes	Yes	3	—	1
		No	1	—	38
	No	Yes	2	—	10
		No	8	71	16

(4) A signal *without* a falling melody form, *without* nasality, but *with* shift should likewise be classified as a pleasure signal,

(5) A signal *without* a falling melody form (usually rising-falling), *without* nasality *and without* shift should be classified as a hunger signal.

The estimated accuracy of this rule is 82 per cent.

Characteristics of the Different Cry Types

For convenience, the information contained in Tables III – XV has been put together in one large table, which forms an appendix (see page 40). On the basis of the information in these tables and the statistical analysis it is now possible to provide a descriptive account of the four cry signals we have been studying, which makes it possible to identify most cry signals of these four types at a glance from the spectrogram. Clearly this should always be confirmed against the rigid criteria set out in the previous section. It is also possible when one is familiar with accounts of the cries and has listened to them on several occasions to identify these four cries literally.

The Typical Birth Signal

The typical birth signal has a length of about one second and its melody form is flat or falling. It is usually voiceless (60 per cent) and always tense. Glottal plosives and vocal fry are rare.

The Typical Pain Signal

The average pain signal is rather long. However, the variation in length is considerable, the standard deviation being 1·5 between 0 and 1 months, and 1·1 between 1 and 7 months. The melody form is usually falling (very rarely rising-falling). The maximum pitch tends to be high and shift is quite often present in about one-third of the cries. Sub-harmonic break occurs in about half the cries and vocal fry in rather more than this. The signals are usually tense. There are no very sharp changes between the first month and the next six months. The length of the cry tends to increase and the maximum pitch to get a little higher. Glottal plosives are less common after the first month, when half the cries have them. Subharmonic breaks become more common.

The Typical Hunger Signal

The melody form of the hunger signal is very characteristic. Over two-thirds of these signals at one month and later have a rising-falling form. The pitch is not very characteristic, although the maximum pitch is lower than the pain signal. Glottal plosives are a characteristic feature and they become commoner after the first month, when two-thirds of the cries have this characteristic. Shift and subharmonic break are rare. There are no very marked changes as the child gets older.

The Typical Pleasure Cry

The typical pleasure cry is often flat in form, and very commonly nasal when this is the case. Its pitch is much more variable than that of the other cries studied and the cries are never voiceless. Cries with shift occur and in these instances the melody form is usually rising-falling. Glottal plosives are rare and the pleasure signals are never tense.

CHAPTER V

Human Identification of the Cry Signals

It has already been shown that the baby's cry can be interpreted correctly by listening to the crying baby (contrary to the opinion of Sherman, 1927) by employing pre-taped birth, pain, hunger and pleasure vocalizations* (Wasz-Höckert *et al.* 1964 a, b, Michelsson *et al.* 1965). Multiple choice testing gives group results well above the pure chance level and shows that experience and training improve the identification ability. Some discrimination has been achieved by a group of physicians and medical students between the cry signals of infants with various pathological conditions and those of normal babies (Partanen *et al.* 1967).

Clearly a series of signals will be easier to identify than single signals but in this study we limited our work to single cry signals alone so that comparison with the spectrographic work was more direct. In fact, as can be seen, results with single signals were very similar to the work with a series of signals.

Identification of the Cries by Observers

The Test Tape

The test items are 24 recorded and selected preverbal cry signals; six from each of the four situational categories described on page 4–7. The items used were selected at random from recordings made in these four situations prior to spectrographic analysis of the data. They were placed in random order on the tape and each cry was repeated seven times with a short interval between each repeat. There was a pause of 5 seconds between each new cry.

Organizing the Testing

The tape was played to 483 adults who were all under the age of 50; 349 were women who had various degrees of experience in child care. They were asked to group each of the 24 signals into one of the given situational categories: birth, pain, hunger and pleasure. Each group was given a standard account of the situation in which the cries had been obtained and what was expected of them.

Results of the Auditory Identification Testing

The results are analysed in: Table XVI (level of performance), Table XVII (errors of different groups of tested persons) and Table XVIII (identifiability of separate test signals).

The test results collected from 349 women have been divided into six groups according to various degrees of experience of child care (Table XVI). The best results obtained were found in the midwife group, mainly because of their outstanding performance in the identification of the birth cry. Children's nurses and mothers follow (the mothers all had one child over 6 months of age) and the remaining (registered

*By vocalization we mean a series of cry signals; usually a series of about 5-10 cries were used.

TABLE XVI

Average performances of female groups in the vocalization test

Group	Total	Birth	Pain	Hunger	Pleasure
		Average amount of right identifications (max. possible in parentheses)			
	(24)	(6)	(6)	(6)	(6)
Midwives (N = 22)	18·2	4·5	4·1	4·8	4·3
Children's nurses (N = 15)	16·8	2·8	4·3	4·7	5·0
Mothers (N = 77)	16·3	3·0	3·8	4·3	5·2
Registered nurses (N = 73)	15·5	2·5	3·9	4·2	4·9
Other women experienced in child care (N = 82)	15·4	2·7	3·7	3·9	5·1
Women with no experience in child care (N = 80)	15·5	2·9	3·6	3·9	5·1
p[1]	< ·001	< ·001	< ·05	< ·001	< ·05

[1]Risk level. Refers to significance between group means (F test).

TABLE XVII

Mean values of P_i and I_i for tested groups

Group	Birth P	Birth I	Pain P	Pain I	Hunger P	Hunger I	Pleasure P	Pleasure I
Midwives (N = 22)	·92	·82	1·12	·62	1·22	·66	·77	·93
Children's nurses (N = 15)	·48	·97	1·22	·59	1·43	·55	·85	·98
Mothers (N = 77)	·62	·81	1·13	·56	1·33	·54	·93	·93
Registered nurses (N = 73)	·53	·78	1·22	·53	1·42	·49	·85	·96
Other women experienced in child care (N = 82)	·60	·75	1·17	·51	1·35	·48	·88	·96
Women with no experience in child care (N = 80)	·65	·74	1·18	·51	1·30	·50	·90	·94

nurses and other women with or without experience in child care) are on about the same level, i.e. 15 correct identifications out of a possible 24, on average. Even the poorest mean (15·4) represents a score that can be obtained by chance in less than one case in a thousand.

A measure of response preference for a particular type of cry for one individual would involve the number of signals the person identified as belonging to this type. Call this total T_i (i = birth, pain, hunger, pleasure). Now $T_i = C_i + W_i$ where C_i is the number of correctly identified type i signals and W_i the number of signals incorrectly identified as type i cries.

As a measure of preference we take

$$P_i = \frac{T_i}{6}$$

since each cry type actually occurs 6 times.

We also define

$$I_i = \frac{C_i}{T_i}$$

which is taken as a measure of identification for type i.

If all the P_i indices for a person are 1·00 this indicates no response preference. If the I_{birth} index is, for example, 0·5 then only half the signals identified as birth signals are in fact birth signals.

TABLE XVIII

Relative frequencies of correct and false situation identifications in the vocalization test. Number of testees = 483.

Situation	*Identification Rank*	*Correct Identifications*	*False Identifications* Birth errors	*Pain errors*	*Hunger errors*	*Pleasure errors*	*Total*
Birth	1	·81		·08	·07	·04	1·00
	2	·65		·26	·08	·01	1·00
	3	·49		·22	·29	·00	1·00
	4	·43		·17	·41	·00	1·00
	5	·32		·41	·28	·00	1·00
	6	·16		·18	·65	·01	1·00
	Mean 1–6	·48		·22	·29	·01	1·00
Pain	1	·76	·06		·18	·00	1·00
	2	·71	·14		·14	·00	1·00
	3	·64	·08		·28	·01	1·00
	4	·63	·07		·30	·00	1·00
	5	·53	·06		·38	·04	1·00
	6	·49	·13		·36	·02	1·00
	Mean 1–6	·63	·09		·27	·01	1·00
Hunger	1	·79	·04	·14		·03	1·00
	2	·74	·03	·20		·03	1·00
	3	·74	·02	·22		·02	1·00
	4	·68	·06	·26		·01	1·00
	5	·61	·05	·33		·01	1·00
	6	·53	·00	·46		·01	1·00
	Mean 1–6	·68	·03	·27		·02	1·00
Pleasure	1	1·00	·00	·00	·00		1·00
	2	·99	·00	·00	·01		1·00
	3	·92	·00	·01	·07		1·00
	4	·84	·01	·05	·10		1·00
	5	·79	·02	·04	·16		1·00
	6	·57	·01	·24	·17		1·00
	Mean 1–6	·85	·01	·06	·08		1·00

For actual empirical figures, see Table XVII. In all tested groups, a preference for pain and hunger responses exists, while there is a lack of preference for birth and pleasure responses. The preferred pain and hunger responses, in terms of being correct or incorrect, are more random than the less preferred birth and pleasure responses, as seen in the lower I-values of the former. One can ask to what degree test performances are due to preferential response patterns. For example, are midwives, by virtue of their professional environment, apt to interpret test signals as birth signals, and if so, to what degree is their performance in the birth scale to be attributed to this preference pattern?

The I-values get smaller in the group series according to mean total scores in Table XVI. Of all the groups, midwives have been most apt to identify signals as birth cries, while the amount of these identifications in other groups is clearly underrepresented in relation to the amount of actual birth signals. In spite of this preference of the midwives, the number of their wrong identification of birth signals is not great (·18). Children's nurses recognized very few birth signals, but ·97 of these identifications were correct.

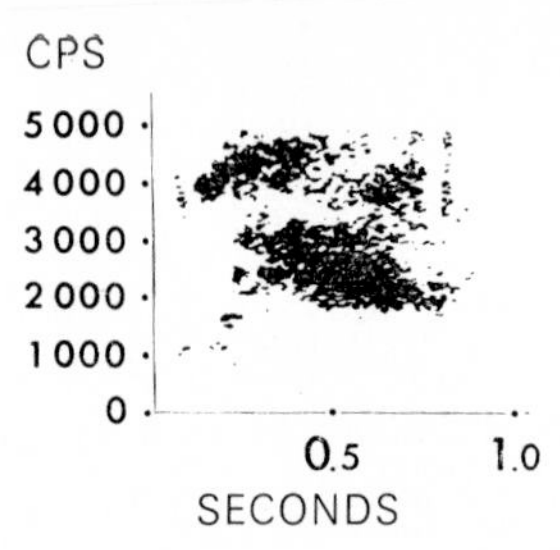

Fig. 19. The best-recognised birth cry.

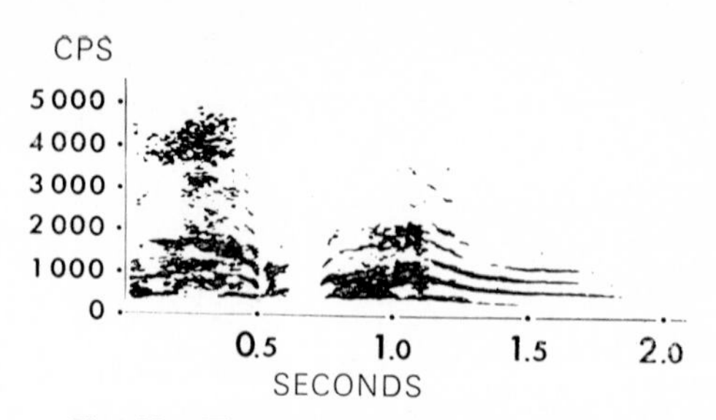

Fig. 20. The poorest-recognised birth cry.

Comparison of the Spectrographic and Auditory Identification

It is of interest to compare the percentages of auditory identification of the 24 cry signals by 483 persons (experienced and inexperienced men and women) with the acoustical attributes obtained spectrographically from these same cry signals.

Birth Cry (6 tested birth cries): Figure 19

This birth cry, recognized by ·81 of the persons tested, is only ·2 seconds shorter than the average of 77 analyzed birth cries, which is 1·1 seconds with a s.d. of ·4 seconds. It is completely voiceless as are ·60 in the reference material. Pitch could not be measured as occurred in most of the voiceless cries. The signal is tense (·94). It has no subharmonic break, nasality, vocal fry or glottal plosives, like the majority of the reference material. Of the subjects, ·08 classified it as a pain cry, ·07 as hunger and ·04 as a pleasure signal.

The poorest recognised birth cry (Fig. 20) was identified by only ·16 of the subjects. It is much longer (1·8 seconds) than the average. It is half voiced, has a very low minimum pitch (270 c/s), (mean: 450 s.d. 60), discontinuous form (·06) with a falling melody. It has been classified as a hunger cry by ·65 of the tested persons, by ·18 as a pain cry, and its attributes suggest that it is indeed somewhat like these cries. Spectrographically it would have been clearly analysed as a birth cry with unusual form.

Pain Cry (6 tested pain cries): Figure 21

The best identified pain cry (·76 made the correct identification) has the following acoustical attributes: length 2·3 seconds, (2·7 and 1·1)*, maximum pitch 740 c/s (680 and 80), minimum pitch 460 c/s (380 and 70), no shift (·17), discontinuous form (·27), no nasality (·75), glottal plosives (·28), no vocal fry (·27) and tense voice (·87). Most of the attributes are very close to the averages for reference material. It has been classified as a hunger cry by ·18 of the subjects and by ·06 as a birth cry. Spectrographically it is not the commonest form of pain cry as it has not vocal fry or melody form, but other features are typical.

The poorest recognized pain cry (identified correctly by ·49) (Fig. 22) has the following attributes: length 2·0 seconds, general pitch 500 c/s, pitch of shift 1510 c/s (incidence of shift in the reference material is ·39), voiced, subharmonic break, falling

*Mean and standard deviation of the reference material.

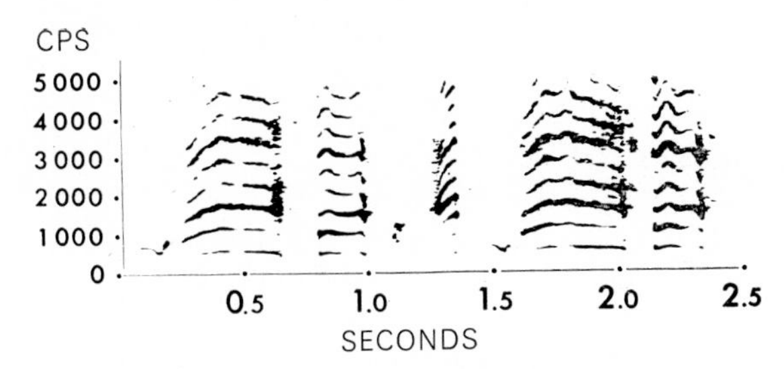

Fig. 21. The best-recognised pain cry.

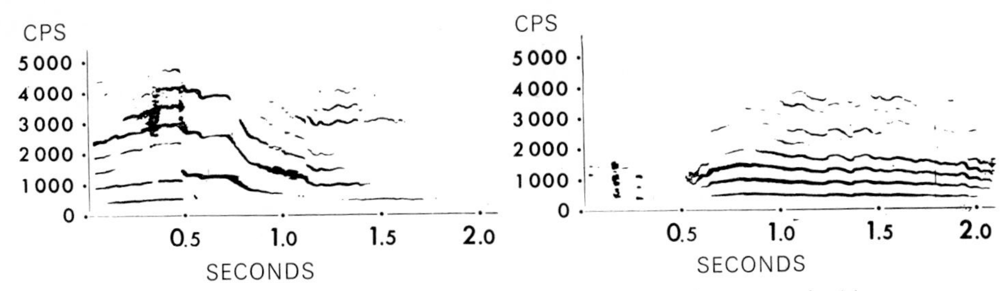

Fig. 22. The poorest recognised pain cry.

Fig. 23. The best-recognised hunger cry.

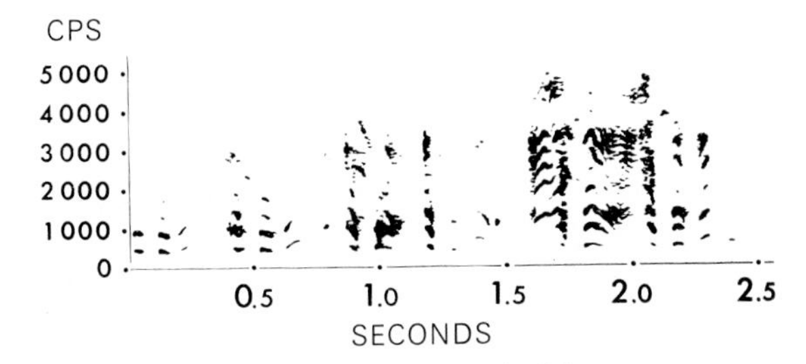

Fig. 24. The poorest-recognised hunger cry.

form (·53), no nasality, no glottal plosives, no vocal fry. ·36 subjects classified it as a hunger cry, ·13 as a birth cry and ·02 as a pleasure cry. However, its acoustical attributes are similar to those of the normal pain cry and its form is more typical than the best recognised pain cry.

Perhaps the occurrence of shift made its identification difficult.

Hunger Cry (6 tested hunger cries): Figure 23

The best identified hunger cry (·79) has the following acoustical attributes: length 1·6 seconds (1·2 and ·6), general pitch 440 c/s (500 and 70), maximum pitch 500 c/s (520 and 80), minimum pitch 360 c/s (420 and 70), no shift, voiced (·68), no subharmonic break (·97), rising-falling form (·81), no nasality (1·00), glottal plosives (·54), vocal fry (·20), lax voice (·58). It was classified as a pain cry by ·14 of the subjects, by ·04 as a birth cry and by ·03 as a pleasure cry. The acoustical features are typical of the reference material.

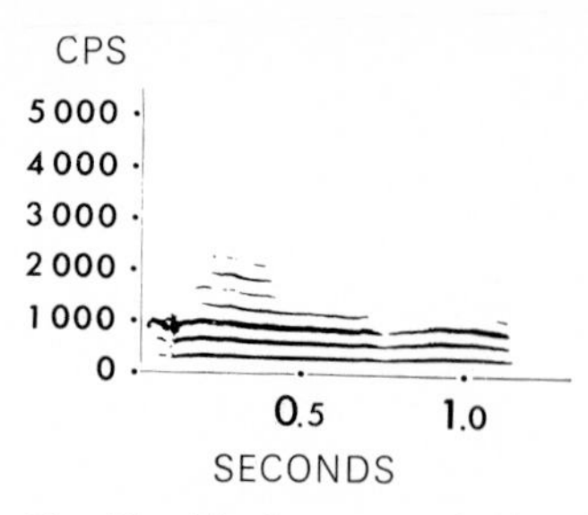

Fig. 25. The best-recognised pleasure signal.

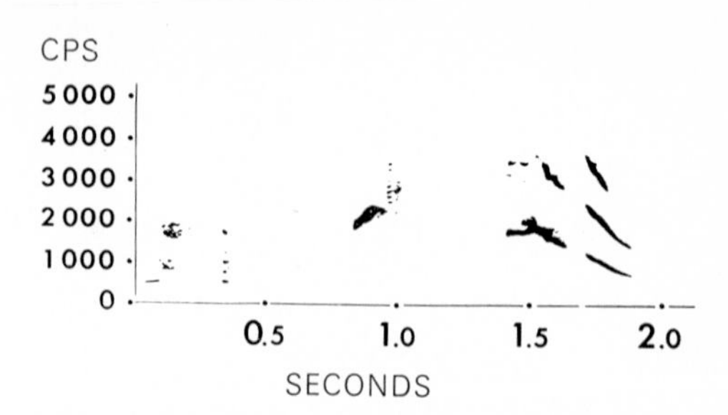

Fig. 26. The poorest-recognised pleasure signal.

The poorest recognised hunger cry (Fig. 24) (identified correctly by ·53) has the following acoustical attributes: length 2·3 seconds, general pitch 490 c/s, maximum pitch 710 c/s, minimum pitch 230 c/s, no shift, half voiced (·23), tense, glottal plosives, no melody form (·14), no nasality or vocal fry. It was classified as a pain cry by ·46 of the tested persons and one can see that it has many attributes in common with a pain cry.

Pleasure Cry (6 tested pleasure signals): Figure 25

The best recognised pleasure signal was correctly identified by all the subjects. It has the following attributes: length 1·1 seconds (1·1 and ·5), general pitch 320 c/s (440 and 90), maximum pitch 350 c/s (650 and 200), minimum pitch 300 c/s (360 and 140), voiced (·76), no subharmonic break (·78), flat form (·46), nasality (·57), no glottal plosives (·90), no vocal fry (·74) and lax voice (1·00). All the attributes correspond closely with spectrographic material.

The poorest recognised pleasure cry (Fig. 26) (·57) has the following acoustical attributes: length 1·8 seconds, minimum pitch 500 c/s, shift with a pitch of 2240 c/s (930)*, voiced, subharmonic break, no melody form (·00), no nasality, glottal plosives, no vocal fry. It has been classified as a pain cry by ·24 of the subjects. Apparently shift and form make the cry difficult to identify. The incidence of shift in pleasure cries is ·19.

The percentages of identification of the different test cries are presented in Table XVIII. The order of mean percentages of correct identification, from the highest to lowest, is: (1) pleasure, (2) hunger, (3) pain and (4) birth signals. Birth signals are often mistaken for hunger (·29) or pain cries (·22). The pain signals have been incorrectly identified as hunger cries (·27) and hunger signals were believed to be pain cries (·27). Errors in identifying pleasure cries are rare.

The range of correct identifications within each signal class (a measure of variability) has been computed and is as follows:

Birth	·65
Pleasure	·42
Pain	·27
Hunger	·27

*The standard deviation has not been computed because of the small number of observations.

These differences appear to reflect the overall acoustical dissimilarity of the test items. The pain and hunger signals appear to have more inner similarity than pleasure and particularly birth signals.

Summary of the Auditory Identification

Experience with infants seems to be of help in infant-adult communication. Experienced groups like midwives, children's nurses and mothers completed the identification test with the best scores. This then is, at least partially, a result of a learning process. The learning mechanism works in such a way that relatively unfamiliar signals are not properly recognised but interpreted in a more familiar framework. Thus all the tested groups except midwives considerably underestimated the number of birth signals in the test tape and identified some of them incorrectly as pain or sometimes hunger signals, which were more familiar to them.

The fact that some signals are more difficult to identify than others holds true *within* signal classes as well. In other words, identification also depends on how representative the signal is of its type. The best identified birth, pain, hunger and pleasure signals therefore also represent spectrographically typical birth, pain, hunger and pleasure signals, and the worst identified signals are in general spectrographically more atypical.

The results also suggest that it should be possible to improve performance by training of those who will care for the child. Preliminary studies with mothers in a Stockholm Maternity Unit have suggested that this may be true. (Greenberg *et al.*, to be published).

CHAPTER VI

Studies of Cries from 'Abnormal' Babies

We embarked on these studies because of an interest in the cry of the normal child and the feeling that his cry signal might give us information about his state which would help us to meet his needs. Nevertheless, an inevitable extension of the technique was to examine abnormal children once we had established the criteria of normality. We believe that the cry can be used as a diagnostic tool in paediatrics (both with 'well' and 'sick' babies). So far, complete analysis of only one condition — the *Cri du Chat* syndrome — has been carried out (Vuorenkoski *et al.* 1966) but our work is sufficiently far advanced with other conditions for us to give some preliminary reports here.

The 'Cri du Chat' Syndrome

One of the problems in studies of abnormal children is to have a clear-cut situation which can be categorised and compared with our normal studies. The easiest situation which the examiner can himself establish is clearly the pain cry, but in some conditions spontaneous cries, which may or may not be associated with pain or hunger situations, may prove most significant. It is the spontaneous cry of some babies (such as in the *Cri du Chat* syndrome) which attracts the attention of the paediatrician. Clearly it is useful to start by analysing what are the features of these babies' cries which alert the doctor. Thus, in *Cri du Chat* it is the spontaneous cry that we have analysed. In analysing the cries the spectrographic analysis was carried out using the same features as in normal studies. The characteristics of the cry are given in Table XIX (44 cries from 8 babies with *Cri du Chat* syndrome). The signals were spontaneous ones and no precise situational category could be assigned. They were compared with both hunger and pain cries.

The typical *Cri du Chat* cry (Fig. 27) was long like a pain cry but variation in length was considerable (2·6 S.D. 1·7). The pitch was invariably higher than that in normal cries and provided an absolute criterion for distinguishing the cry from normal ones. Melody form was often flat or rising, which rarely occurs in pain or hunger states. The cries were voiced, tense and rarely contained glottal plosives. There were two distinctive features of the cry: (1) inspiratory cries of 70·4 sec. which are rare in normal infants* and (2) the similarity of the signal in inspiratory and respiratory signals makes them difficult to separate and there is no clear 'on—off' phenomenon as occurs normally.

Down's Syndrome

Since the diagnosis of Down's syndrome can be established so firmly with chromosome studies this is clearly a very interesting group of abnormal babies to examine in

*They do not occur in ordinary pain or hunger cries. We have only seen them when 'normal' babies have been left unattended for a long period after the start of a pain or hunger cry and appear 'desperate'. There may, of course, be other situations when they arise which we have not studied.

TABLE XIX

Means, medians and percentages of different variables in normal hunger and pain signals and spontaneous signals from children with maladie du cri du chat.

Attribute	*Normal Material* Pain cries (60)	Hunger cries (75)	*Cri du Chat* 8 *Babies* 44 *Cries*
Length, sec.	2·7	1·2	2·6
Standard deviation	1·1	0·6	1·7
General pitch, cps.	530	500	860
Standard deviation	80	70	165
Maximum pitch, cps.	680	520	1030
Standard deviation	80	80	200
Minimum pitch, cps.	380	420	750
Standard deviation	70	70	165
Occurrence of shift, %	83	—	—
Pitch of shift, cps.	910	—	—
Occurrence of subharmonic break, %	62	3	9
Rising-falling, %	18	81	5
Falling, %	77	0·4	16
Rising, %	0·2	—	23
Flat, %	0·3	0·1	54
Falling-rising, %	—	—	2
No form, %	—	14	—
Occurrence of vocal fry, %	75	20	—
Occurrence of tenseness, %	87	42	95
Dichotomous singal, %	—	—	23
Expiration-inspiration signals, %	—	—	18
Voiceless signals, %	8	9	—
Half-voiced signals, %	20	23	16
Voiced signals, %	72	68	84

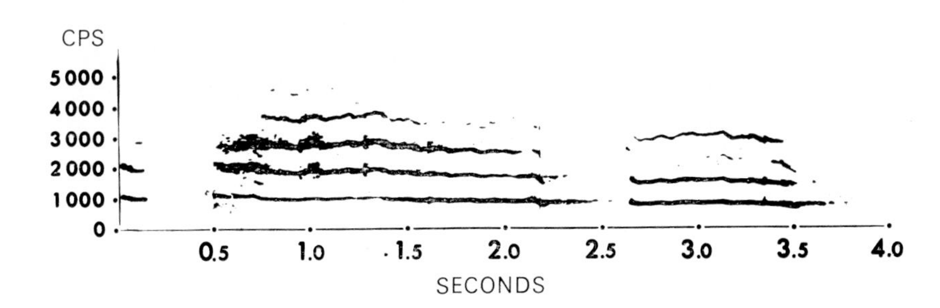

Fig. 27. Typical spontaneous cry in a baby with Maladie du Cri du Chat. For details of spectographic analysis see text.

crying situations. Many detailed studies of Down's syndrome have been made (see, for example, Penrose 1966), but little attention has been drawn to the characteristics of the cry (Karelitz *et al.* 1960, Fisichelli *et al.* 1966). Down's syndrome babies do not have strikingly distinct spontaneous cries like the *Cri du Chat* syndrome babies. We have analysed cries collected in pain situations (Fig. 28) which prove to have quite distinctive features, and it is possible to train observers to identify Down's syndrome cries by 5 minutes' work with a test tape. Spectrographically the pain cries of Down's syndrome children present the following features. The typical melody form is flat, rather similar to that of the spontaneous *Cri du Chat* signals, but the cries are of low pitch, lower even than the pain cries of normal infants. The cry is tense and often only half voiced. Spectrographically it is difficult to identify the features of this tenseness which distinguishes the cry from normal pain cries, but this is undoubtedly one of the features which make auditory identification possible. Periodically on the spectrogram the tenseness is heightened (when attacks of glottal 'pressure' are superimposed on the phonation). Normal pain cries are never long, of low pitch and flat in form at the same time and these babies are therefore very easy to pick out on cry analysis. We have studied three babies in whom a diagnosis of Down's syndrome had been entertained but spectrographically the cry was not typical of Down's syndrome and chromosome analysis confirmed this finding. Two cases were seen where again the diagnosis of Down's syndrome was in some doubt, but here the spectrographic analysis of the cry was typical of Down's syndrome and on chromosome analysis both these babies proved to have the condition. It is therefore likely that spectrographic analysis, which gives a quick diagnosis, will be a useful supplement to chromosome analysis. Our report on Down's syndrome will be appearing shortly (Lind *et al.* 1968).

'Brain Damaged' Children

We have studied a number of children who received a cerebral insult in the perinatal period and were causing concern to the paediatricians supervising them (see Lind *et al.* 1965). Clinical details on these babies are not fully available as they have not been followed up for a long enough period, but some of them have clear subsequent evidence of brain damage while others have recovered. At the time that they were examined spectrographically they were 'in difficulties'. None of them suffered from any other defects such as Down's syndrome.

Auditorily the cries were not as easy to identify as Down's Syndrome or *Cri du Chat* cries but sometimes the observer was struck by them. The cries tended to be short and rather shrill and they sounded as if two separate phonations were going on at the same time. Spectrographically the analysis confirmed these features. The curious double phonation is shown in Figures 29 and 30, the melody form is variable but the pitch is high and the signal is typically short. The phonation is very erratic and the signal may be discontinuous. It has considerable variations in pitch. Detailed analysis of these cries has not yet been carried out but a preliminary look at the data suggests that cry analysis may well help in deciding on the extent of the neurological involvement in infants who have suffered a perinatal insult.

Our work on other types of abnormal cries is in a preliminary state (Partanen *et al.* 1967) but in Figures 31-35 we show examples of cries with abnormal acoustical features which we have collected from babies who clinically had also been assessed as 'abnormal'.

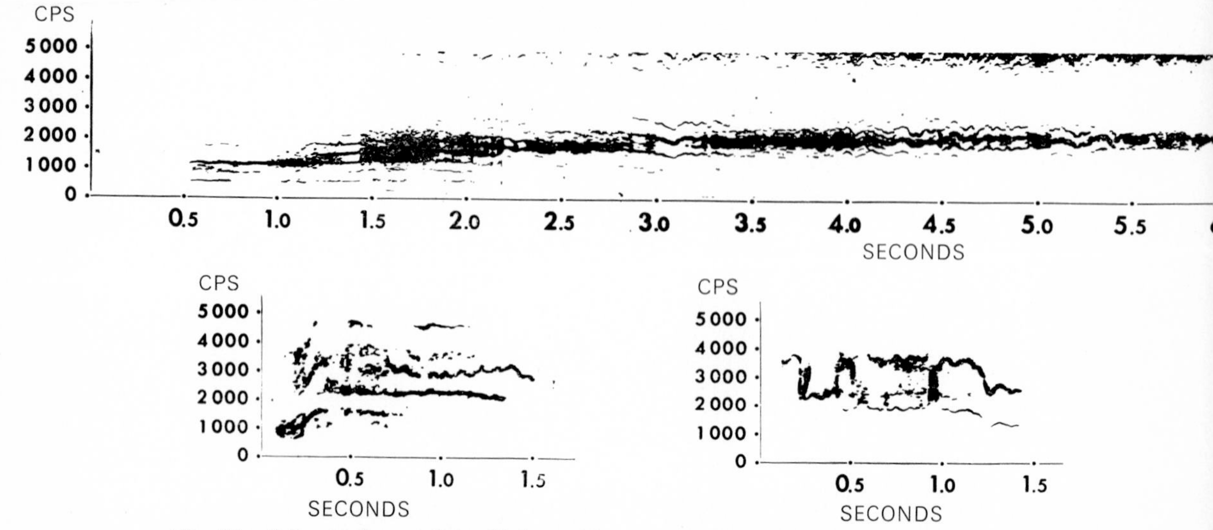

Fig. 29. Pain cry from a baby (2 days old) with a clinical diagnosis of asphyxia neonatorum and 'brain damage'. Note the double phonation at 0·7—1·4 seconds.

Fig. 30. The same baby one day later. The cry has different features to Fig. 29 but the double phonation is still present.

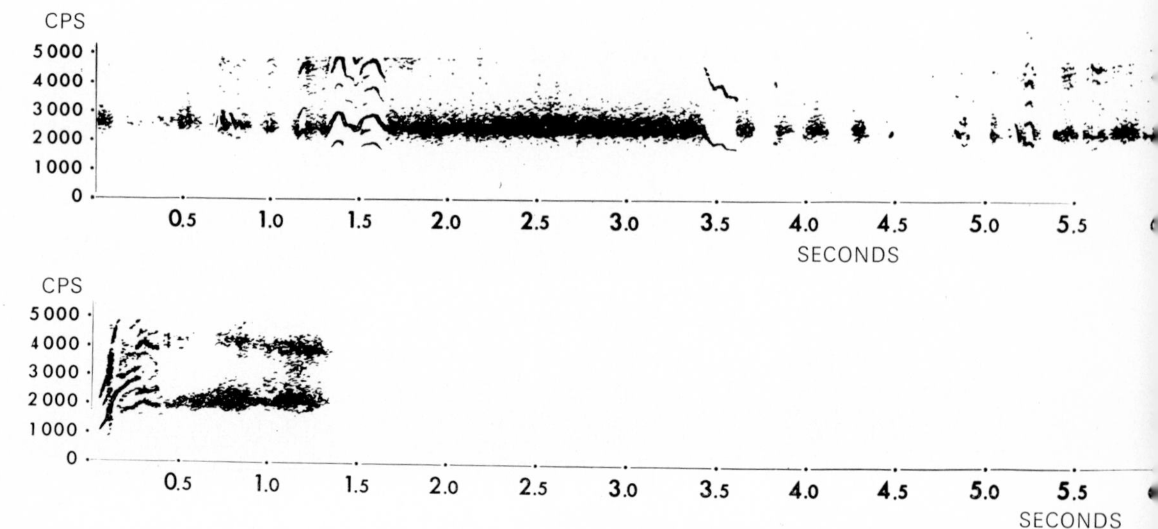

Fig. 33. Another very long discontinuous signal from a baby with 13/15 triso

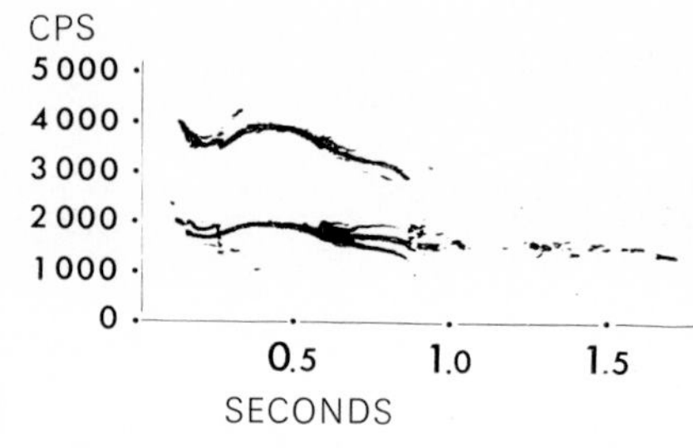

Fig. 34. Pain cry from a baby whose serum bilirubin was 23 mg. on day 2 and who had an exchange transfusion immediately following the recording of this cry. The phonation breaks up in a curious way at 0·6 seconds. This phenomenon has only been found in hyperbilirubinaemia. This baby's subsequent development was normal.

Fig. 28. Pain cry in a baby with Down's syndrome. For details of spectographic analysis see text.

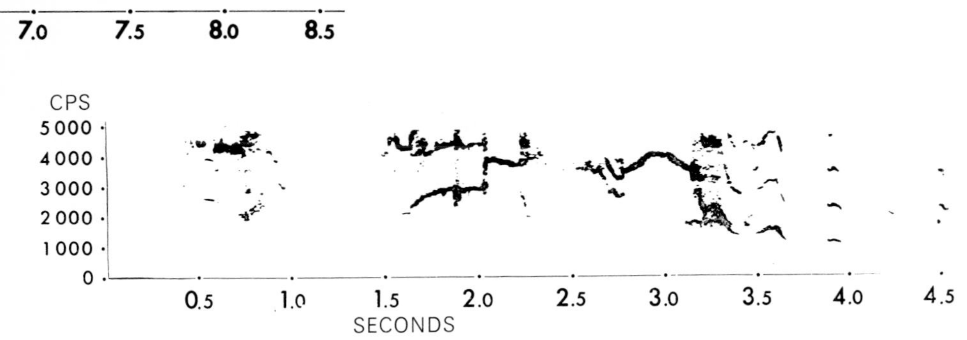

Fig. 31. Pain cry in a newborn infant who breathed poorly, probably as a result of drugs given to the mother one hour before delivery. The baby had two cyanotic attacks on the first day of life but his subsequent history was uneventful. This is a typical pain cry of a baby with asphyxia neonatorum but no brain damage. 14 hours old.

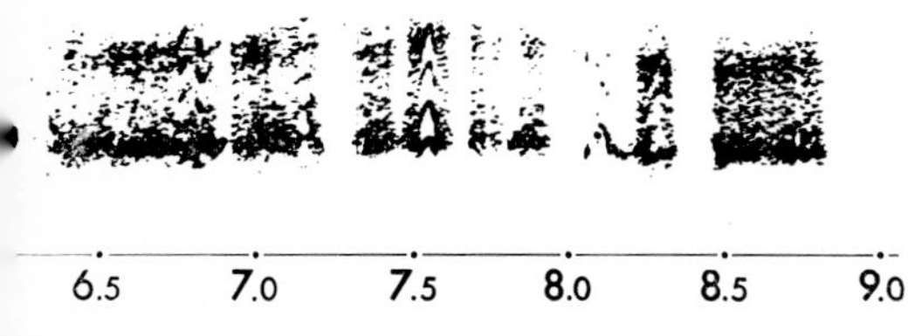

Fig. 32. Pain cry in a baby who developed meningitis in the newborn period. The sustained, strident phonation is a feature of this cry.

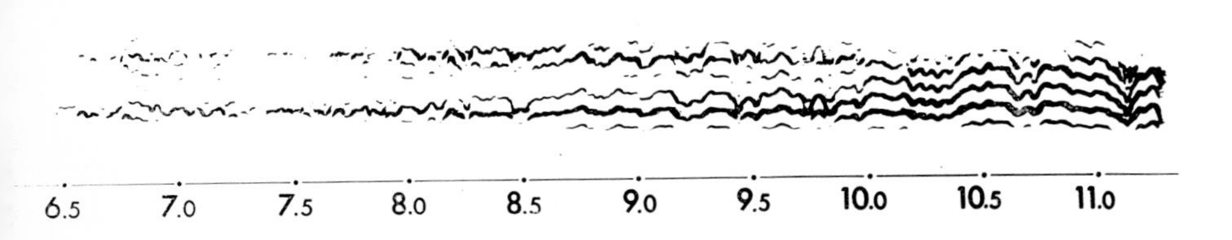

re are similarities with Down's syndrome cries.

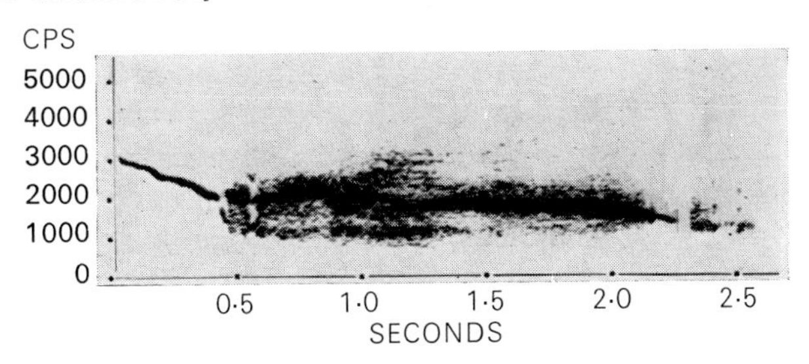

Fig. 35. Pain cry from a baby with congenital internal hydrocephalus. Note the marked shift at the beginning of the cry.

CHAPTER VII

Value of Cry Studies

Our hypothesis was that cry signals in young infants were significant and our results demonstrate that this is the case. In our view the study of the cry has two important implications:

1. *Normal Children.* The doctor in the past had no basis for his advice to parents about the nature of the child's crying. His advice has been based on the fads and fancies of the day. Mead and Newton (1967) have commented validly on this situation and draw attention to different culture patterns in different parts of the world. As they remark 'Most primitive peoples respond immediately to the fussing infant, giving some kind of personal interaction, usually the breast. Western observers record with amazement how quiet and 'good' many primitive babies appear to be.' They quote Spock (1957), who says 'If a baby has been crying hard for 15 minutes or more and if it's more than two hours after the last feeding — or even if it is less than 2 hours after a *very small* feeding — give him another feeding. If it's less than 2 hours after a full feeding, it's unlikely that he's hungry. Let him fuss or cry for 15 or 20 minutes more.' Illingworth and Karelitz are among the few paediatricians who have paid serious attention to the problem of crying. We are not yet able to say that we can always identify the meaning of the baby's cry, but we can say that crying in newborns is purposive. The baby is trying to communicate with the adult and it would be churlish not to respond. So far we have only identified four situations, (1) the cry of the baby who is in pain, (2) the cry of the baby who is hungry, (3) the pleasure cry and (4) the birth cry. We hope, however, that we shall in time identify other patterns. We believe, for example, that sometimes babies require handling and gentle movement (which is known to be essential for the development of some other mammals) and it is possible that the need is communicated by a specific signal. Scientific study of this nature is the way in which the paediatrician of the future should handle the problems of the mother and her young baby. Early developmental patterns appear to relate to the child's future developmental behaviour, and therefore adequate movement of the normal young child may have profound effects on the individual's whole future life.

2. *Abnormal Children.* Analysis of the cry signal is a valuable addition to the newborn neurological examination. Standard paediatric tests frequently mention abnormal cries which are sometimes stated to be characteristic for particular syndromes. However, it has rarely been possible to provide an adequate verbal description of the cry and there are relatively few situations where the pathognomic nature of the cry has been firmly established (an example is the *Cri du Chat*). It now seems likely that there are many instances where spectrographic examination of the cry will provide valuable additional information. Clinical conditions where we think the cry will prove of value

include cerebral insult following birth traumas (anoxia and haemorrhage), kernicterus and newborn hypoglycaemia, hydrocephalus, meningitis and intercranial haemorrhage. For example, in kernicterus, the cry signal is of particular interest owing to the well known fact that the level of serum bilirubin does not reflect closely the presence or absence of a cerebral involvement. As the cry signal originates in the central nervous system it is reasonable to suggest that together with other items in the newborn examination it will provide more information about the state of the brain than studies of blood levels of significant metabolites.

At the present time we are studying three main groups of infants: (1) babies with chromosomal anomalies, (2) babies with other congenital anomalies, (3) babies at risk of cerebral injury or involvement.

Future Acoustical Studies

It will be useful in the future to relate cry studies to all the usual biological variations. Genetic, psychological, environmental and cultural factors are no doubt all important but we have not studied many of them yet. From the genetic point of view, Ostwald *et al.* (1962) studied the vocalisation of infant twins. They showed that the cries of monozygotic twins are more similar than those of dizygotic twins but their reported work was in a preliminary phase. The possible influence of the sex on the character of the cry in our study has so far given negative results. We have done some work on infant cries both in South America and Japan and believe that babies' cry signals are culturally free and represent a truly international language, although further work is needed to confirm this hypothesis.

Acoustical Features of the Cries we have Studied

The interpretation of the birth cry is complicated and some marked differences among signal types can be seen in this period. When considering the newborn situation during the birth process one might wonder if the birth cry was a pain signal. However, the typical birth cry, when compared with the pain cry after birth, has distinctive features. It is similar in general pitch and tenseness, but birth signals differ from pain signals in length and type of melody and in their maximumum and minimum pitch.

The pain cry, as we have suggested, is the procedure which is easiest to use as a clinical test as it is the easiest to standardise. We have used two different types of stimulation, pinching and vaccination, and while in future we intend to use only one, we have not observed a significant difference between pain cries resulting from different forms of stimulation. We interpret these results as an indication that both stimuli produced the maximal cry reaction. It is probably the tenseness of the cry in the baby which is partly responsible for the discomfort felt by the listening adult (see Ostwald 1963) and which produces the drive to relieve the infant's needs. This especially affects the mother (Sullivan 1953).

The hunger cry is the most open to question of those we have studied, because it is difficult to be certain that the baby's cry *is* because he is hungry. It has been interesting to note, however, that the characteristics of the hunger and pain cries are distinct, although we have sometimes observed pain cries being given by a baby who has been hungry for a long time. In the studies reported here the hunger cries were always collected before the noon feed and the babies had always been fed some four hours earlier. We have, however, collected hunger cries from babies before the morning feed and in some instances these infants had not been fed for some seven hours. We were interested to note in these tapes many cry signals which more nearly resembled typical pain cries than hunger cries.

Developmental Course of Cries

Changes in the characteristic features of the signal types can be seen during the first 3 — 5 days after birth. Of the 13 acoustical attributes measured, four seem to show clearcut tendencies in this period. The flat melody type tends to disappear and the incidence of glottal plosives increases. Shift disappears completely but vocal fry increases. These changes occur in hunger cries during the first 3 — 5 days of life. These changes in the hunger cry may represent the establishment of the hunger situation itself. After the 5th or 7th day changes become less marked although there is a tendency for the increase of glottal plosives throughout the newborn period. Pain cries during the same period show the opposite tendency with the incidence of glottal plosives decreasing.

After these early days it is interesting to note that changes in the acoustical attributes of the cries studied are not observed throughout the remaining 7 months in which we have collected cries. This is not the case with the pleasure signal, which from the 5th month of age onwards shows increasing variability. This is undoubtedly when the child is beginning to experiment with his utterances and emits sounds which are the precursors of real speech, although the relationship between these early babbling sounds and speech is not a simple one.

Auditory Identification of Personal Characteristics of Cry

Throughout this study we have emphasised the value of auditory study of the cry signals as well as spectrographic studies. There is no doubt the two can assist each other. There are presently certain limitations to the spectrographic technique. For example it has not been possible to distinguish spectrographically one baby's isolated cry from another's. It has been shown, however, that mothers are able to identify their own babies' cries during the neonatal period from a test tape which included 8 other babies' cries (Valanne *et al.* 1967). This has also been shown in an interesting study by Formby (1967) and these studies indicate that the cry has individual and personal characteristics. Not all mothers were able to identify their baby's cries in the newborn period and in addition some cries from babies who were normally recognised by their mothers were unrecognisable. It is, therefore, difficult to decide which cries and which features of the cry are significant for this personal identification. Where the mother cannot identify the baby's cry it is impossible to tell whether the fault lies in the baby or the mother and this will be so until we can evolve spectrographic techniques for identifying personal characteristics.

Illingworth and Parviainen (1949) have drawn attention to intrauterine crying. There is a mythology surrounding this subject. It was believed that intrauterine crying foretold the birth of great men. Napoleon and Mahomet are among those reported to have let forth these prenatal sounds. However, although man appears to have believed in the importance of crying from the earliest times, the incomprehensibility of the signal (and possibly the vanity of great men) has meant that little attention has been paid to them in the past. Now, however, that we begin to understand their nature we believe that the study of the infant cry will achieve the significance it deserves.

Appendix

TABLE A

Means, medians and frequencies of different attributes in the groups of birth, pain, hunger and pleasure signals

Attribute	0-1 *Months* *Birth* (77)	*Pain* (60)	*Hunger* (74)	P*	1-7 *Months* *Pain* (60)	*Hunger* (74)	*Pleasure* (72)	P*
Length, sec. (mean)	1.1	2·6	1·3	< ·001	2·7	1·2	1·1	< ·001
(s.d.)	0·4	1·5	0·6		1·1	0·6	0·5	
General pitch, cps (mean)	500	530	470	< ·001	530	500	440	< ·001
(s.d.)	60	80	40		80	70	90	
Max. pitch, cps (mean)	550	650	550	< ·001	680	520	650	< ·001
(s.d.)	70	100	60		80	80	200	
Min. pitch, cps (mean)	450	410	390	< ·001	380	420	360	< ·05
(s.d.)	60	90	60		70	70	140	
Occurrence of shift	·18	·32	·04	< ·01	·38	—	·19	< ·001
Pitch of shift, cps (median) **	870	1140	***	< ·05[2]	910	—	930	<N.S.**
Voice quality:								
Voiceless signals	·60	·07	·20	< ·001	·08	·10	—	< N.S.**
Half voiced signals	·35	28	·20		·20	·23	·24	
Voiced signals	·05	65	·60		·72	·68	·76	
Signals with Subharmonic break	·03	·48	·10	< ·001	·62	·03	·22	< ·001
Melody form;								
Rising-falling	·13	·23	·78		·18	·81	·31	
Falling	·31	·62	·01		·77	·04	·10	
Rising	·03	·08	—	<·001	·02	—	·08	<·001
Flat	·36	·02	·11		·03	·01	·46	
Falling-rising	—	—	—		—	—	·06	
No form	·16	·05	·09		—	·14	—	
Nasal signals	·05	·18	·11	< ·05	·25	—	·57	< ·001
Glottal plosives:								
No glottal plosives	·79	·50	·50	< ·001	·72	·31	·90	< ·001
Glottal plosives	·21	·50	·37		·28	·54	·10	
Only glottal plosives	—	—	·13		—	·15	—	
Signals with vocal fry	·04	·63	·28	< ·001	·73	·20	·26	< ·001
Tense signals	·94	·90	·42	< ·001	·87	·42	—	< ·001

P* = risk level, determined by using the usual χ^2 and F tests. See also next footnote.

** Because of the small number of observations and some skewness in the pitch of shift distributions, medians have been used in the description, and the nonparametric Mann-Whitney U method in testing the significance of the differences between pitch of shift of birth and pain signals (0—1 m.), and pain and pleasure signals (1—7 m.). Hunger signals are thus omitted. For description of the Mann-Whitney U test, see Siegel (1956).

*** not calculated.

References

Aldrich, C. A., Sung, C., Knop, C. (1945) 'The crying of newly born babies. I. The community phase. II. The individual phase. III. The early period at home.' *J. Pediat.*, **26**, 313, **27**, 89, 428.

Allport, G. W. (1960) Personality: A Psychological Interpretation. London: Constable.

Berry, M. F., Eisenson, J. (1956) Speech Disorders. New York: Appleton-Century-Crofts.

Bosma, J. F., Lind, J., Truby, H. M. (1965) 'Distortions of upper respiratory and swallow motions in infants having anomalies of the upper pharynx.' *in* Lind, J., ed., Newborn Infant Cry. *Acta paediat. Scand.*, Suppl. 163.

——, ——, —— (1965) 'Studies of neo-natal transition: correlated cineradiographic and visual-acoustic observations.' *in* Lind, J., ed., Newborn Infant Cry. *Acta paediat. Scand.*, Suppl. 163.

Brazelton, T. B. (1962) 'Crying in infancy.' *Pediatrics*, **29**, 579.

Bühler, C. (1930) The First Year of Life. New York: Day.

Fairbanks, G. (1942) 'An acoustical study of the pitch of infant hunger wails.' *Child Develop.*, **13**, 227.

Fisichelli, V. R., Karelitz, S. (1963) 'The cry latencies of normal infants and those with brain damage.' *J. Pediat.*, **62**, 724.

—— Haber, A., Davies, J., Karelitz, S. (1966) 'Audible characteristics of the cries of normal infants and those with Down's Syndrome'. *Perceptual and Motor Skills*, **23**, 745.

Formby, D. (1967) 'Maternal recognition of infant's cry.' *Develop. Med. Child. Neurol.*, **9**, 293.

Friedhoff, A. J., Alpert, M., Kurtzberg, R. L. (1962) 'An effect of emotions on voice.' *Nature* (*Lond.*), **193**, 357.

——, ——, —— (1964) 'An electroacoustical analysis of the effect of stress on voice.' *J. Neuro-psychiat.*, **5**, 266.

Gabriel, K. R. (1964) 'A procedure for testing the homogeneity of all sets of means in an analysis of variants.' *Biometrics*, **20**, 459.

—— (1966) 'Simultaneous test procedures for multiple comparisons on categorical data.' *J. Amer. stat. Ass.*, **61**, 1081.

Gesell, A. (1940) The First Five Years of Life. New York: Harper.

Greenberg, M., Vuorenkoski, V., Partanen, T. J., Lind, J. (1967) 'Behavioural changes and cry patterns in the first two hours of life in early and late clamped newborn.' *Ann. Paediat. Fenn.*, **13**, **64.**

——, Lind, J., Rosenberg, I. 'An evaluation of primiparous mothers from rooming-in and conventional units: a study of the effects of rooming-in in Sweden.' To be published.

Hurlock, E. B. (1950) Child Development. New York: McGraw-Hill.

Illingworth, R. S. (1955) 'Crying in infants and children.' *Brit. med. J.*, **i**, 75.

—— (1957) The Normal Child. London: Churchill.

Irwin, O. C. (1952) 'Speech development in the young child. II. Some factors related to the speech development of the infant and young child.' *J. speech Dis.*, **17**, 269.

Jakobson, R., Fant, G., Halle, M. (1952) Preliminaries to Speech Analysis. M.I.T. Technical Report, No. 13.

Joppich, G. (1964) 'Uber die Entwicklung der Sprache.' Nestle Ag. Dgg 006841. (Recorded lecture in German.)

Kaplan, H. M. (1960) Anatomy and Physiology of Speech. New York: McGraw-Hill.

Karelitz, S., Karelitz, R., Rosenfelt, L. (1960) 'Infants' vocalisations and their significance.' *in* Bowman, P., Mautner, H. (Eds.) Mental Retardation, Proceedings of the International Conference on Mental Retardation, 1959. New York: Grune & Stratton. p. 439.

—— Fisichelli, V. R. (1962) 'The cry thresholds of normal infants and those with brain damage.' *J. Pediat.*, **61**, 679.

Kyttä, J. (1964) 'Finnish oesophageal speech after laryngectomy, sound spectrographic and cineradiographic studies.' *Acta Otolaryng.*, Suppl. 195.

Landtman, B., Wasz-Höckert, O., Vuorenkoski, V. (1964) 'The use of sound spectrography in pediatric cardiology.' *Ann. Paediat. Fenn.*, **10**, 122.

Lanyon, W. E., Tavolga, W. N. (1960) 'Animal sounds and communication.' *in* Proceedings of the A.I.B.S. Symposium at Bloomington, Indiana, 1958. Washington.

Lind, J. (ed.) (1965) Newborn Infant Cry. *Acta paediat. scand.*, Suppl. 163.

—— Wasz-Höckert, O., Vuorenkoski, V., Valanne, E. (1965) 'The vocalisation of a newborn brain damaged child.' *Ann. Paediat. Fenn.*, **11**, 32.

——, ——, ——, Partanen, T., Theorell, K., Valanne, E. (1966) 'Vocal response to painful stimuli in the newborn and young infant.' *Ann. Paediat. Fenn.*, **12**, 55.

—— Vuorenkoski, V., Rosberg, G., Partanen, T. J., Wasz-Höckert, O. (1968) 'Spectrographic analysis of vocal response to pain stimuli in infants with Down's Syndrome.' To be published.

Lynip, A. (1951) 'The use of magnetic devices in the collection and analysis of the preverbal utterances of an infant.' *Genet. Psychol. Monogr.*, **44,** 221.
McKusick, V. A. (1958) Cardiovascular Sounds in Health and Disease. Baltimore: Williams and Wilkins.
Mead, M., Newton, N. (1967) 'Cultural patterning of perinatal behaviour.' *in* Richardson, S.A., Gutimacher, A.F. (eds.) Child Bearing. Its Social and Psychological Aspects. Baltimore: Williams and Wilkins. Edinburgh and London: E. and S. Livingstone.
Michelsson, K., Vuorenkoski, V., Partanen, T., Valanne, E., Wasz-Höckert, O. (1965) 'Identifikation av spädbarnets preverbrala Kommunikation.' *Finska Lakaresallsk. Handl.*, **109,** 43.
Miller, G. A. (1951) Language and Communication. New York: McGraw-Hill.
Minnigerode, B. (1963) 'Klinische und vergleichend-anatomische Untersuchungen zur Erzeugung der hohen Schrilltöne menschlicher Säuglinge.' *Arch. Klin. Exp. Ohr. Nas. Kehlkopfheilk.*, **181,** 208.
Osgood, C. E. (1953) Method and Theory in Experimental Psychology. New York: Oxford University Press.
Ostwald, P. F. (1963) Soundmaking. Springfield, Ill.: C. C. Thomas.
—— (1964) 'Acoustic manifestations of emotional disturbance.' Disorders of Communication, **42,** 450.
—— Freedman, D. G., Kurtz, J. H. (1962) 'Vocalisation of infant twins.' *Folia Phoniat.* (*Basel*), **14,** 37.
Palva, T. (1958) 'Whispered voice audiometry.' *Acta Otolaryng.*, **49,** 531.
Partanen, T. J., Wasz-Höckert, O., Vuorenkoski, V., Theorell, K., Valanne, E., Lind, J. (1967) 'Auditive identification of pain cry signals of young infants in pathological conditions and its sound spectrographic basis.' *Ann. Paediat. Fenn.*, **13,** 56.
Parviainen, S. (1949) 'Vagitus uterinus.' *Ann. Chir. Gynaec. Fenn.*, **38,** 330.
Penrose, L. S., Smith, G. F. (1966) Down's Anomaly. London: Churchill.
Potter, R., Kopp, G. A., Green, H. C. (1947) Visible Speech. New York: van Nostrand.
Prechtl, H., Beintema, D. (1964) The Neurological Examination of the Full-Term Newborn Infant. London: Spastics Society Medical Education and Information Unit/ William Heinemann Medical Books.
Ringel, R. L., Kluppel, D. D. (1964) 'Neonatal cry: a normative study.' *Folia Phoniat.* (*Basel*), **16,** 1.
Sedláckovà, E. (1964) 'Analyses acoustiques de la voix des nouveau nés.' *Folia Phoniat.*, **16,** 44.
Sherman, M. (1927) 'The differentiation of emotional response in infants.' *J. comp. Psychol.*, **7,** 335.
Siegel, S. (1965) Nonparametric Statistics for the Behavioural Sciences. New York: McGraw-Hill.
Spitz, R. A., Cobliner, W. G. (1965) The First Year of Life. New York: International Universities Press.
Spock, B. (1957) The Common Sense Book of Baby and Child Care. New York: Meredith.
Sterling, T. S., Pollack, S. V. (1965) Computers and the Life Sciences. New York: Columbia University Press.
Sullivan, H. S. (1953) The Interpersonal Theory of Psychiatry. New York: W. W. Norton.
Trojan, F. (1957) 'General semantics'. *In* Kaiser, L., ed., Manual of Phonetics. Amsterdam: North Holland.
Truby, H. M., Lind, J. (1965) 'Cry sounds of the newborn infant.' *in* Lind, J., Ed. Newborn Infant Cry. *Acta paediat. Scand.*, Suppl. 163.
Valanne, E., Vuorenkoski, V., Partanen, T. J., Lind, J., Wasz-Höckert, O. (1967) 'The ability of human mothers to identify the hunger cry signals of their own newborn infants during the lying-in period.' *Experientia*, **23,** 768.
van Riper, C. (1954) Speech Correction: Principles and Methods. New Jersey: Prentice-Hall.
Vuorenkoski, V., Lind, J., Partanen, T. J., Lejeune, J., Lafourcade, J., Wasz-Höckert, O. (1966) 'Spectrographic analysis of cries from children with maladie du cri du chat.' *Ann. Paediat. Fenn.*, **12,** 174.
Wasz-Höckert, O., Partanen, T., Vuorenkoski, V., Valanne, E., Michelsson, K. (1964a) 'Effect of training on the ability to identify specific meanings in newborn and infant vocalisations.' *Develop. Med. Child Neurol.*, **6,** 393.
——, ——, ——, ——, —— (1964b) 'The identification of some specific meanings in newborn and infant vocalisation.' *Experientia*, **20,** 154.
——, Valanne, E., Vuorenkoski, V., Michelsson, K., Sovijärvi, A. (1963) 'Analysis of some types of vocalisation in the newborn and in early infancy.' *Ann. Paediat. Fenn.*, **9,** 1.
——, Vuorenkoski, V., Valanne, E., Michelsson, K. (1962) 'Tonspektrographische Untersuchungen des Säuglingsgeschreis.' *Experientia*, **18,** 583.
——, ——, ——, ——, Lind, J. (1964c) 'Estudios espectrográficos de los gritos de hambre en los recién nacidos e infantes.' *Rev. mex. Pediat.*, **33,** 98.